INTERMITTENT FASTING
FOR WOMEN
OVER 50

D1712564

GET FIT AND FORGET ABOUT HUNGER STRIKES
WITH A TAILORED FASTING PLAN, 150+
HEALTHY RECIPES, AND A WEEKLY OMAD
PLAN TURN BACK THE CLOCK AND FEEL LIKE A 30YO

Brenda Pylon

Table of Contents

Introduction

Intermittent fasting is an eating practice that alternates between fasting and eating times. In other words, you should eat only at a given period. This type of diet doesn't specify what food to eat, but when to eat it. The point here is to say that, in the true sense of the word, periodic fasting or Intermittent Fasting (IF) is not a diet.

Periodic hunger is a practice in the course of human evolution. Supermarkets, refrigerators, or food were not available throughout the year for ancient people. They were not able to find anything to eat at times. As a result, people have evolved to function for long periods without food. Indeed, occasional fasting is more natural than ever eating 3-4 (or more) meals a day.

Anyone serious about lifting weights, exercise, and living a healthy lifestyle knows that the best way to build muscle mass and an aesthetically shaped body is to eat healthy foods and drink lots of protein.

But to build lean muscle mass is not enough. Nobody in the world can build muscles without losing fat. To remove the fat while making sure you don't lose muscle mass, you need to change your diet. This change is referred to as regular fasting. You should achieve this goal with this eating pattern. One study shows that periodic fasting or Intermittent Fasting (IF) causes less muscle loss than standard diets with limited calories.

Intermittent fasting (IF) is a dietary pattern that alternates between periods of hunger and a reduced diet, resulting in weight loss and better overall health.

The most common reason people use this form of "periodic fasting" is weight loss. This diet will cause you to eat less. This can lead to an involuntary decrease in the consumption of calories. This, in effect, results in a loss of weight. Of course, it all depends on you. For the rest of the time, you shouldn't overdo it.

For an extended period, when you have not eaten food, the body begins to look for other energy sources. The first option it uses is in the form of glycogen and fat-stored carbohydrates. Regular fasting well planned, reduces glycogen and burns fatter. If you do your workout for the day at the end of your fasting, you're going to burn even more fat. For instance, if you haven't eaten anything since 6:00 p.m. the night before, you go to the gym at 8:00 a.m. fasting the following day and then your first meal at 10:00 a.m. you're doing 16 hours of daily fasting. This is the most popular method, as described above.

Periodic fasting or intermittent fasting (IF) will increase your metabolism marginally while allowing you to eat fewer calories. This is a very effective way of weight loss and fat burning.

Intermittent fasting may appear to be a good option for women who want to lose weight, but many wonder if women should fast. Is intermittent fasting beneficial to females? A few key studies on this program have been published, and they can help shed some light on this fascinating new dietary trend.

Intermittent fasting has some advantages for women. The fact that females have a much higher fat proportion in their bodies makes it especially important for ladies trying to lose weight, an activity when the body burns carbohydrate stores for the first 6 hours before switching to fat burning. Fasting is a viable option for women struggling with stubborn fat despite following a healthy diet and exercise plan.

CHAPTER 1

As the name suggests, intermittent fasting consists of alternating periods of normal balanced eating, and short periods of fasting. The fasting periods are often between 12 and 16 hours; the "skipped" meal can be breakfast or dinner depending on your preference. Fasting enthusiasts mainly use it to lose weight, whether during a dry period for bodybuilding enthusiasts or when they simply want to shed pounds.

This program includes alternating periods of eating and fasting in which you may eat as much as you like during the eating window but only drink water during the fast. The goal is to achieve the calorie reduction benefits and use it as a tool to lose weight.

Intermittent fasting can be done over several days, alternating 24-hour cycles or hourly. The first option requires abstaining from some or all meals one or more days of the week. Daily fasting involves 24 hours feeding and fasting cycles that start at the same time every day, e.g., fast from Monday 6 pm to Tuesday 6 pm; eat as much as you like from Tuesday 6 pm to Wednesday at 6 pm; repeat the process. There is a short period of eating during the occasional intermittent fasting, usually 4-6 hours within the 24-hour day during which you can consume as much as you like.

Some of the facts that put people off are the fear of being extremely hungry and not sticking to the plan or understanding how to fit it into your schedule. This is quite easy if you plan to eat your evening meal pretty much at the same time every day, but either side at an hour depending on whether you're doing an intermittent fasting or eating process. You can also handle socializing and dining out with a little preparation yet again.

Today, the most common IF protocols include fasting for 16 hours each day and restricting food intake to one or two days each week. If you consider intermittent fasting a normal part of the human eating pattern, then it can be said that humans are designed to implement it. Our hunter-gatherer ancestors probably did as well. Under this new plan, individuals who engage in planned intermittent fasting could potentially benefit their health in multiple ways, such as increased body composition, longer life span, and reduced aging.

INTERMITTENT FASTING AFFECTS WOMEN AND MEN DIFFERENTLY

While men may find intermittent fasting easier than women, there is some evidence that it may not be as beneficial for some women as it is for men.

When it comes to blood sugar control, it was found that women were negatively impacted after three weeks of intermittent fasting. However, men were not.

Some women claim that after starting intermittent fasting, their menstrual cycles have changed.

Such changes occur because female bodies are extremely sensitive to caloric restriction. When calorie intake is low, such as fasting for too long or frequently, the hypothalamus is affected.

The secretion of GnRH, a hormone that helps to release two reproductive hormones: LH and FSH can be interrupted (FSH).

Without a clear connection between the hypothalamus and the ovaries, it is difficult to determine whether you

have regularly or irregularly timed periods, infertility, poor bone health, and other health problems.
While some researchers believe that fasting may result in a reduction in the size of the ovaries and disrupted reproductive cycles in rats, other researchers are skeptical of this claim and think that just a few weeks of alternating fasting reduces ovary size and irregular cycles in rats. Although human studies do not confirm the animal testing results, several additional types of scientific studies have validated the conclusions of these investigations.
For these reasons, women should consider using a modified approach to intermittent fasting, such as having fewer days, as well as shorter periods of fasting.

HOW INTERMITTENT FASTING WORKS?

Fasting essentially allows the body to use stored energy, such as consuming excess body fat.
It is vital to understand that this is normal and that humans have adapted to move without having to suffer adverse health effects. All energy from the food

is contained in body fat. If you don't feed, the body can actually' use' its fat for energy.
Life is about equilibrium: the good and the bad.
By consuming more food, more energy than we can use is absorbed. Some of that energy needs to be retained for later use. Insulin is the principal hormone involved in the production of food energy.
This helps to store excess sugar when consuming insulin in two different ways. Sugars in long chains can bind glycogen, which is then stored in the liver. Nevertheless, storage space is small and once it is full, the liver begins converting excess glucose into fat. This cycle is called de novo lipogenesis (which means "re-creating fat").
Some of the newly created fat is retained in the liver but most of it is transferred to other body fat stores. Though this process is more complicated, the amount of fat produced has no limit. The body has two compatible feeding energy storage mechanisms. One is very easy to access, but it has a limited storage capacity (glycogen) and the other is the hardest to reach. Still, it does have an unlimited storage capacity (body fat.)
The cycle works in reverse when we don't eat (fasting). Insulin levels drop, allowing the body to start burning stored energy since it no longer receives food. Glucose in the blood drops, and the body must pump glucose from the tank to use it as fat.
Glycogen is energy's most open source. It breaks down into glucose molecules to provide energy to other cells. In this way, enough fuel can be supplied to the body for 24-36 hours. Instead, the body begins to break down to use fat as fuel.
The body can only be in two states: absorption (high insulin) and fasting (low insulin). Either we store the food energy, or we waste energy. It's one procedure or another. If there is a balance between eating and fasting, then there is no net weight gain.
When we begin to eat from the moment we get up and don't stop until we go to sleep, we spend most of the time in the state of absorption. We'll gain weight over time. We left no time to burn food energy to the body.
To restore balance or lose weight, we simply need to increase the time we consume food energy. It is fasting.

Fasting allows the body to use stored energy. After all, that is what it is about. You need to remember that nothing is wrong with this: that is how the body is designed. It's what dogs, cats, tigers, and bears do and we humans do.
When you eat regularly, as is often advised, the body uses the fuel from the food that comes in and does not consume the body fat, it will only store it. The body keeps it for when there is nothing to eat.

Many investigations have studied the effects of intermittent fasting on the human body in some of its modalities. More research is needed but the results are very promising: intermittent fasting causes blood insulin levels to drop, particularly after 16 hours of fasting, making it easier to burn fat and increase the growth hormone that builds muscles, strengthens the immune system, and regenerates joints. Short-term fasting induces autophagy in the brain, a mechanism by which neurons kill their harm.

Restricting the amount of food in worms and rats, which can live twice as much, has shown to prolong life. It seems that intermittent fasting works the same way but without a miserable life of constant hunger. Fasting activates sit-ins, proteins that control inflammation and aging, protects cells from oxidation and prevent cancer cells' proliferation.

Intermittent fasting tends to increase insulin sensitivity, reducing glucose levels, and thus could be used to avoid type 2 diabetes.

The diet has been proven effective in reducing inflammation and oxidative stress, two of the trigger factors of cardiovascular disease.

Intermittent fasting decreases LDL cholesterol, raises cholesterol from HDL, reduces blood pressure and triglycerides, avoiding worse problems. It has succeeded in stopping Alzheimer's disease in rats. Also, nine of ten participants improved in a recent trial with human patients, thanks to the fasting program.

How to do it

It may not be easier to test the effects of intermittent fasting personally, but keep in mind these indications:

• Most of the fasting time at night is the most comfortable way. For example, the day you start, you usually eat at noon, and you no longer eat during the day. Skip breakfast the next day and eat at noon for the first time.

• Drink water as if tomorrow wasn't there. You can also drink tea, coffee, and any liquid with no calories in general. It's not allowed to add honey to the tea.

• Start with a day of weekly fasting. For instance, if you acclimatize well on Tuesday and Friday, you can do it on two non-consecutive days.

• It is recommended that the day you start fasting should be a day off from your workout program. The next day's trend, exercise just before the first meal.

• Avoid prolonged fasting exercise. Take a small portion of protein, a shake, or amino acid tablets containing leucine if you exercise strength or intervals, so you stop burning muscle mass.

TYPE OF INTERMITTENT FASTING

METHOD 16/8

The process consists of 16-hour fasting and the remaining 8-hour eating period during which you can eat normally.

This method suits most routines very well because of its practicality. But it only becomes an effective tool if you apply it the right way.

To be successful, mix the time you are sleeping with the time of your fast. Generally, at least that's what is recommended, your sleep should be 8 hours long.

So, it's been 8 hours of fasting without any effort. Now, if you are used to skipping your breakfast and eating only for lunch, it is very likely that you will easily adapt to the 16/8 method.

For example, suppose you have dinner at 8 pm and sleep there at midnight. So far, it's been four hours of fasting.

If you wake up at 8 am, skip your breakfast and have lunch at noon, you will finish at 4 pm fasting without any problem.

People who don't like breakfast or who don't like it are the ones who benefit most from this method. But even you who are not used to it can try. Sometimes it's just a matter of getting used to it.

24-HOUR FAST

It requires 24 hours of fasting once or twice a week. If you are a beginner, this type of fasting can be difficult. You need to be very well prepared because a whole day without eating is a challenge that requires a lot of body resistance.

No solid food can be eaten during fasting. Everything that has a considerable caloric value-greater than 20 Kcal-should be avoided.

Drink only water, tea, or coffee without sugar, or sweeteners. After your 24-hour fast, you can go back to eating as usual.

Before fasting, try to consume foods that contain plenty of protein and fiber so that you are fuller during the fast.

This is a great method for those who want to extend the benefits of autophagy-the process of cell renewal. That's because it takes longer periods to occur and brings significant effects to your health.

Rejuvenation, increased longevity, cancer prevention, and treatment are some of the benefits of cell autophagy. Anyway, if you are already adapted to intermittent fasting-withstand 24 hours of fasting-and want to enjoy the benefits of cell regeneration, 24-hour fasting is a very interesting option.

PROTOCOL 5: 2

The 5: 2 protocol is a modified version of the 24-hour fast. If it gets to be about one to two whole days of fasting, on those days it is allowed to consume a small number of calories.

The number of days you can fast remains the same. The only change is that you can now consume some calories on fasting days.

For women, around 500 Kcal per day is recommended. Men are recommended 600 Kcal daily.

Take great care with your food content and pay close attention to the way you distribute your calories throughout the day.

Give priority to foods that offer you a prolonged feeling of satiety.

In this way, instead of eating poor foods that may soon satisfy you, you are extending the duration of your fast and, consequently, receiving more benefits.

It is worth mentioning that if you divide your calories into small portions and consume them between short periods, for example, every 3 hours, the insulin spikes will diminish the full benefit of the benefits of fasting.

Try to have a maximum of two meals of 250 Kcal if you are a woman or two meals of 300 Kcal if you are a man. The time of these meals is up to you.

Beginners interested in fasting for 24 hours, even knowing their difficulty, should try this type at least once. It is much more flexible and promotes significant weight loss.

ALTERNATE FASTING DAYS

As the name suggests, alternating fasting days boil down to taking turns between fasting days and regular feeding days. That is one day of fasting, one day of eating, and so on, consecutively.

In the original model, you cannot consume anything other than liquids without calories. But other, more malleable versions break some of that constraint.

There are people who on fast days consume 25% (1/4) of their caloric needs. Others consume about 500 Kcal during fasting.

As previously stated, depending on how the calories are used, it is also much easier to practice alternating fasting days and enjoy their benefits.

Its main benefits are: great weight loss, decreased insulin resistance, more longevity, and heart health.

If you want to lose weight for an event that is close to happening, this method can help you stay in shape.

However, it is a model that, if followed as proposed by the standard version-24 hours of fasting-is extremely difficult to remain in the long term.

This depends on your body's adaptation to this type of eating pattern.

ONE DAILY MEAL

People, who love to test their limits, whether physical or mental, often eat a daily meal.

Currently, it is one of the most severe variations that exist. That's because you only have one hour to eat. The remaining 23 hours are done on an empty stomach.

The good thing is that there is a great incentive for you to eat healthy and complete foods since you only have one hour to meet your needs and prepare yourself again for another long journey.

Plus, you don't have to worry about what time you need to eat or how many meals you should eat.

Those who for some reason are having a very busy day can take advantage of this method.

Eating a single meal every day is much easier since you are adept at the ketogenic diet.

The ketogenic diet changes your metabolism and, as it is based on higher consumption of healthy fats; you have more energy to perform your tasks.

Although a daily meal can provide some benefits, it is quite laborious to maintain such a model for a long time.

WARRIOR'S DIET

Developed by writer Ori Hofmekler, the warrior's diet consists of 20 hours of fasting and 4 hours of food.

It is possible to consume some foods derived from milk, such as cheese and yogurt, vegetables, fruits, and boiled eggs during fasting. But they must be consumed in small quantities.

For the remaining 4 hours, you eat as much as you want. The author advises the consumption of natural and healthy products.

Although the foods suggested by Hofmekler have low concentrations of carbohydrates, if consumed in large amounts, they can break your fast.

The absence of limits makes the warrior's diet imprecise and arbitrary. Recommending eating a little something does not say what the exact amount is.

Even a fruit is capable of interrupting your fast, which slows down its speed of reaching ketosis. Remember that ketosis is the main cause of the benefits of intermittent fasting.

Therefore, some people are successful and others are not. Only those who calculate their macronutrients or those with luck in their favor receive benefits in this style.

But don't get discouraged. If you follow a diet, such as the ketogenic, which restricts and counts your car bo-hydrates, the warrior diet can help you lose weight, increase your energy and concentration.

ABSOLUTE FASTING

For some people, it is very uncomfortable to go for long periods without eating. Now, imagine if they could not drink water or any other liquid during fasting.

Wouldn't it be sad? Yeah, well! This is how absolute fasting works. You simply choose the type of fast that meets your needs, the only restriction being not drinking water while you are fasting.

This certainly makes absolute fasting one of the most—if not the most—radical types of intermittent fasting.

His followers believe that water scarcity accelerates three times the speed to achieve some benefits of fasting. This is the case with weight loss in which, due to the lack of water, hydrogen atoms are removed from the fat to form H_2O molecules. As a result, you would burn more fat.

But so far there is no scientific evidence to prove whether this process occurs and, if it does, at what speed. Furthermore, running out of liquid can put your life in danger. This is because the volume of water produced through fat is not sufficient to maintain its vital functions.

So, before trying a type like this, visit your doctor or nutritionist and check that there are no other more viable alternatives.

Best Types of Intermittent Fasting for Women Over 50

There is no one-size-fits-all strategy when it comes to dieting. This refers also to extended fasting.

In general, women should approach fasting more relaxed than men.

This could include shorter fasting times, fewer days of fasting, and eating a limited number of calories on fasting days.

Here are some of the best forms of female intermittent fasting:

• Crescendo method: fast from 12 to 16 hours for two or three days a week. Fasting days should be non-consecutive and evenly distributed throughout the week (e.g., Monday, Wednesday, and Friday).

• Eat (also called 24-hour protocol): a total fast of 24 hours once or twice a week (maximum twice a week for women). Start with fasts for 14 to 16 hours and gradually increase.

• Diet 5: 2 (also called "Quick Diet"): limit calories to 25% of the usual consumption (about 500 calories) for two days a week and eat "normally" for the other five days. Allow one day between fasting days.

• Modified fasting on alternate days: fasting on alternate days, but eating "normally" on days without fasting. It is allowed to consume 20 to 25% of the normal calorie intake (about 500 calories) on a fasting day.

• The 16/8 method (also called the "Lean gains method"): fast for 16 hours a day and eat all calories in an eight-hour window. Women are advised to start with a 14-hour fast and finally up to 16 hours.

Whatever your choice, during non-fasting periods, it is still essential to eat well. During the eating window, if you consume many unhealthy, high-calorie foods, you may not experience the same weight loss and health benefits.

The best approach is the one you can tolerate and sustain in the long run, which does not have adverse health consequences.

CHAPTER 2

BENEFITS OF INTERMITTENT
FASTING OVER 50

HEART HEALTH

Heart disease is the number one cause of death in the world. In turn, high blood pressure, high LDL cholesterol, and elevated triglyceride concentrations are some of the biggest risk factors for developing that condition.

A research of 16 overweight men and women found an elevated rate that reduced blood pressure by 6 percent in just eight weeks after following a fasting program.

Intermittent fasting in the same study decreased LDL cholesterol by 25% and triglycerides by 32%.

Nevertheless, the association between intermittent fasting and increased LDL cholesterol levels and triglycerides is not reliably clear.

Higher-quality studies with stronger methods are needed before researchers can fully understand the effects of intermittent fasting on heart health.

DIABETES

Intermittent fasting can also help manage and effectively reduce the risk of diabetes.

Some of the risk factors for diabetes appear to be reduced by intermittent fasting compared with extended caloric restriction.

This is done primarily by raising insulin levels and increasing insulin resistance.

In a randomized controlled study of more than 100 overweight or obese women, six months of intermittent fasting resulted in a 29% reduction in insulin levels and a 19% reduction in insulin resistance. There was no change in the blood sugar levels.

Besides, it has been shown those 8 to 12 weeks of intermittent fasting decreases insulin levels by 20 to 31 percent and blood sugar levels by 3 to 6 percent in people with prediabetes, a disorder in which blood sugar levels are normal, but elevated just enough to diagnose diabetes. Nevertheless, intermittent fasting may not be as beneficial for women in terms of blood sugar as it is for men.

A small study showed that blood sugar regulation decreased for women after 22 days of fasting in alternating days, while men had no adverse effect on blood sugar. Because of this side effect, decreasing insulin and insulin resistance will probably reduce the risk of diabetes, especially in patients with pre-diabetes.

WEIGHT LOSS

Intermittent fasting can be an easy and effective way to lose weight if done correctly, as regular short-term fasting can help you consume fewer calories and lose pounds.

Several studies suggest that intermittent fasting is as effective for short-term weight loss as conventional calorie-restricted diets.

A study of overweight adult research in 2018 showed that intermittent fasting resulted in an average weight loss of 6.8 kg (4 pounds approximately) over a 3 to 12-month period.

Another study found that intermittent fasting over 3 to 24 weeks in overweight or obese adults decreased body weight by 3 to 8 percent. The study also showed that participants decreased their waist diameter by 3–7 percent during the same period.

It should be recalled that the long-term effects of intermittent fasting on weight loss for women have not yet been shown.

In the short term, intermittent fasting appears to help you lose weight. However, how much you lose depends on how many calories you eat during times without fasting, and how long you stick to the lifestyle.

It Can Help to Eat Less

Switching to intermittent fasting can help you eat less naturally.

One study found that when their food intake was restricted to a four-hour window, young men consumed 650 fewer calories per day.

Other Health Benefits

Several studies in humans and animals suggest that intermittent fasting may also produce other health benefits.

• Reduction of inflammation: some studies show that intermittent fasting can reduce the main inflammation markers. Chronic inflammation can lead to weight gain and some health issues.

• Psychological well-being improvement: one study found eight weeks of intermittent fasting reduced depression and compulsive eating behaviors while improving obese adults ' body image.

• Longer life: it was shown that intermittent fasting extended the shelf life of rats and mice by 33–83 percent. The impacts in lifespan on humans have not been determined yet.

• Preservation muscle mass: intermittent fasting tends to be more effective than constant calorie restriction in maintaining muscle mass. A higher muscle mass, even at rest, makes you burn more calories.

• Reduction of insulin levels. This is rational because high levels of insulin hinder the release of accumulated body fat. When insulin levels are not quickly lowered, the body will not obtain energy from accumulated body fat.

• According to this study, the sensitivity of insulin increases when a person fasts intermittently. If the insulin sensitivity is low, the insulin cells in your body are not responding well. Insulin resistance is a factor that contributes to type 2 diabetes and also promotes fat storage.

• Increment in your body's growth hormone: This induces the release of body fat and encourages muscle growth.

• Weight loss: You'll lose weight with normal calorie limits and intermittent fasting. Intermittent fasting though may increase the likelihood of muscle preservation by shredding body fat. Research and the personal results of Martin Berkhan indicate that intermittent fasting preserves a higher proportion of lean mass, rather than a daily caloric deficit.

• Cognitive effects: the increase in catecholamine fasting may positively affect the concentration and focus of the mind. You can also work for a long time, without worrying about food intake. These two elements can combine to boost your productivity.

• Decreased risk for heart disease. Coronary heart disease is one of the leading causes of death among men and women worldwide.

• Promotion of neuronal autophagy: Neuronal autophagy is the process of cells recycling waste materials and rebuilding themselves. Your brain's functions depend largely on neuronal highways. Eliminate this cycle and your brain won't do well.

• Rapid increase of BDNF levels (Brain-derived neurotropic factor): It fosters the formation of new neurons and synapses. Alzheimer's disease is associated with low BDNF rates and the rise of BDNF has neurological benefits to combat Alzheimer's disease.

- Ketosis: There may be sporadic ketosis. This is a system in which the body absorbs energy from stocks of fat. This sets off the keto.

PSYCHOLOGICAL BENEFITS OF INTERMITTENT FASTING

- Increased ability to concentrate: from an evolutionary point of view, it is possible to think that after eating, certain cognitive functions are impaired. This is to be expected since after eating, the sympathetic nervous system necessary to start cognitive functions is deactivated and the parasympathetic is activated. Also, studies indicate that during fasting the levels of neurotransmitters associated with the psychological state of concentration increase, such as norepinephrine and orexin.
- Enhancement of neuroplasticity, the brain's ability to create new connections: Entering ketosis and alternating between the different ways of obtaining energy stimulates brain plasticity.
- Protection against depression. There is a substance produced by the brain, BDNF (brain-derived neurotrophic factor) that is almost absent in depressed people. Boosting its production protects from depression. This can be enhanced by intermittent fasting.
- Protection against inflammatory processes: Inflammatory processes can interfere with the functioning of the nervous system. Faced with this condition, the body allocates its resources to fight inflammation and subtract cognitive functions. So, if we reduce the inflammation of the body performing periods of fasting, we encourage those resources to be allocated to what is necessary.
- Reduction of food craving: It helps us recognize hunger and satiety signals, assisting us in avoiding emotional or boredom hunger.
- Reduction of mental fatigue. The way we eat, especially if ultra-processed foods are included in our diet, produces insulin spikes responsible for mental fatigue. If after fasting we eat natural or "good processed" foods, these peaks are reduced.

DISADVANTAGES OF INTERMITTENT FASTING

There is no perfect way of example that also applies to extend fasting. Of course, to be efficient with this system, you also need to consider certain drawbacks from the very outset. Unless you feel you can survive without games, then you're mistaken. The fasting time is only half as adequate without strength training and supplementary endurance activities. There's nothing in here, even without a predominantly healthy diet. Occasionally junk food is permitted, but it may not be scandalous. So, with that principle, you don't get a free pass to celebrate.

While it has a positive effect on most aspects of life, there are some notable downsides to take into account. Being conscious about the deficiencies of IF will help you make better decisions and possibly go several hours without consuming food, especially if you are used to eating several times a day.

To a much greater extent, especially in the early stages, the threat of abandoning is exceptionally great for those who enjoy feeling the epigastrium's discomfort, also known as the hunger pain. Conversion might increase the likelihood of a relapse.

Intermittent fasting is not appropriate for those who have already overcome an acute eating disorder because it may lead to a new eating disorder. People with diabetes, because of the abrupt and substantial decrease in blood sugar levels, are not advised to go on an extended fast.

As an original form of human nutrition, fasting at intervals is not far from our internal conditioning. Consequently, the potential for weight loss success is excellent. The method works; and that has already been demonstrated by hundreds of thousands of people. If you want to get rid of annoying body fat effectively and mentally rely on this nutritional form, you should give a fasting interval opportunity.

ADVANTAGES OF FASTING COMPARED TO DIETING

ADVANTAGE ONE: IT'S SIMPLE

Lack of consensus about what constitutes a healthy diet also creates patient uncertainty. Is there a low-fat diet they should be on? Down with carbohydrates? Under-calorie? Down with sugar? Low on the glycaemic index? A radically different fasting approach makes it easier to understand. Two sentences suffice to describe it. Nothing to sleep. Drink water, tea, bone broth, or coffee.

That's all, diets can fail because of ineffectiveness, but also because they're not properly followed up. The most obvious advantage of fasting is its simplicity, which is the main reason for its effectiveness. The easier the better when it comes to the dietetic laws.

ADVANTAGE TWO: IT'S FREE

Of course, in an ideal world, everyone would eat organic vegetables and organic beef that had grazed near them instead of white bread or highly processed food. The fact remains that, sometimes, these organic foods will cost up to 10 times more that of industrial food.

The government subsidizes cereals, making them far more competitive than other foods. For this reason, a kilo of cherries can cost € 8 or € 9 while a baguette is worth about € 1 and even less a packet of pasta. Feeding a family of pasta and white bread over a tight budget is much simpler.

No matter how efficient a scheme is when its costs are prohibitive. The price makes it unaffordable for those who can afford it. This should not allow them to have type 2 diabetes and its limitations.

Fasting is free. In reality, it doesn't just cost zero, it saves you money as you don't have to buy food at all! No expensive goods. No overpriced food supplement. No meal substitute or medicine. It's gratis.

ADVANTAGE THREE: IT'S PRACTICAL

Eating uncooked raw foods on your own is good for your health. Most people, however, have neither the time nor the inclination to make food every day. Time is the center of work, education, family, children, extracurricular activities, and personal activities. Cooking takes time: shopping, preparing the meal, without forgetting the time to cook and the time to clean it all. It takes time for everything, and time is a scarce commodity that is usually sorely lacking.

Even if it is with the best intention in the world, advising everyone to cook isn't the best strategy if you really want to get results. Fasting, by contrast, is the exact opposite: more shopping, more preparation ingredients, cooking, and cleaning. It's a way of simplifying your life. Fasting itself is convenient. Nothing to do. Many schemes give directions. Fasting needs nothing. Keeping it easier is hard!

ADVANTAGE FOUR: YOU CAN ENJOY THE LITTLE PLEASURES OF LIFE

Many diets recommend making the ice cream or dessert a definite cross. That's certainly good advice to lose weight. But putting it into practice is not easy. It goes on to abstain for six months or a year, but what about your remaining days? And then, why do you want to? Think a little over it. What could be more fun than sharing the assembled piece at your best friend's wedding and toasting with a glass of champagne? Want to abandon those pleasures forever? Instead of a birthday cake, choose a birthday salad? Existence loses its flavor a little bit, isn't it? There's a long time to live.

Fasting after occasional sprains helps restore balance. That is the essence of the cycle of life. Abundance carries on from drought. Starvation causes overflowing. It was always this way. Since time immemorial, feasts have always been celebrated with birthdays, weddings, parties, and other special occasions.

Nevertheless, such feasts must be accompanied by fasts. You can afford deviations by not eating as soon as you compensate them. Fasting is above all about equilibrium.

ADVANTAGE FIVE: IT'S POWERFUL

Many people with type 2 diabetes are considered overweight and have marked insulin resistance. Sometimes even a strict ketogenic diet (very few carbohydrates, not too much protein, and lots of fat) is not sufficiently powerful to cope with the condition. Fasting is the easiest and most effective way of reducing insulin and improving insulin resistance in those situations. Fasting is powerful to conquer the stages during weight loss and raising the need for insulin.

The number of fasts that can be performed is not limited, and this is the main therapeutic benefit. The longest reported fast has lasted 382 days, with no detrimental effect on the patient. If it often happens that the fast doesn't yield the expected results, it's enough to increase the frequency or length until the target is achieved. By the way, diets—low in fat, low in carbohydrates (low carb,) or paleo—work for some people but not others. If you don't get any diet results, you'll have little leeway to make it more effective. On the other hand, with fasting, you just need to lengthen the time! The faster you go, the more likely you will lose weight, but it will always happen.

ADVANTAGE SIX: IT'S FLEXIBLE

Many diets recommend starting to eat in the morning, and then splitting meals by consuming the rest of the day every two-and-a-half hours. For some people, that type of diet works well. Nevertheless, finding and preparing something to eat six, seven, or eight times a day is extremely difficult. However, it is possible to go for 16 hours or 16 days at any time. There is no set deadline. You can fast one day a week, 5 days the next week, then 2 days the next. Fasting adapts to your responsibilities and enables several durations to be combined without being locked into a system.

If you live in the United States, the Netherlands, the United Arab Emirates, the polar Arctic desert, or Saudi Arabia's sandy desert, you can fast everywhere. Fasting makes your life simpler once again because you just have nothing to do. Where other proposals add complexity, it brings simplicity. If you don't feel well at some point in the fast, simply stop fasting. The malaise is going to go away.

ADVANTAGE SEVEN: IT IS COMPATIBLE WITH ALL DIETS

The compatibility of fasting with all diets is its big asset. It does not impose any particular practice but, on the contrary, it consists of doing nothing.

- Are you not eating meat? This isn't stopping you from fasting.
- Are you not eating wheat? This isn't stopping you from fasting.
- Do you have an allergy to the dried fruit? This isn't stopping you from fasting.
- Short-term? This isn't stopping you from fasting.
- Are you running short? This isn't stopping you from fasting.
- Are you always on the go? This isn't stopping you from fasting.
- You're not sure how to cook? This isn't stopping you from fasting.
- Are you eighty-five years old? This doesn't deter you from fasting.
- Do you have difficulty chewing? This isn't stopping you from fasting.

Not eating for 16 hours is the trend: Intermittent fasting is the new miracle weapon for healthy and sustainable weight loss. Besides, the intermittent avoidance of food should inhibit inflammation in the body and lower blood pressure. A temporary hype or a sensible form of nutrition? Here you get the facts.

The intermittent fasting principle is explained in a few words: You do not consume food for 16 hours - except for water, unsweetened teas, and even black coffee. Drinking a lot is even a must. You can eat normally for the remaining 8 hours. There are no restrictions. Whether you skip breakfast or (late) dinner is also up to you.

If you eat food, it is broken down into its components and released into the bloodstream. If your food contains carbohydrates, your blood sugar level will also rise. To regulate this, your body releases more insulin to transport the sugar molecules from the blood to the cells needed (e.g., brain, heart, muscles). As long as blood sugar and insulin levels are elevated, your cells prefer to use sugar for energy. The fat burning then runs to a minimum.

If you forego food, the opposite is the case: blood sugar and insulin remain stable and your body increasingly relies on existing fat deposits. This increases your fat metabolism and relieves the digestive system. Other advantages: Interval fasting can inhibit inflammation, lower blood pressure, and promote new brain cells. Incidentally, it is not a new "invention". In the past, when people still had to get their food by hunting and gathering, they were used to long meal breaks and the body "optimized" for them.

Incidentally, intermittent fasting can help you lose weight sustainably and without the yo-yo effect. The prerequisite: a negative energy balance. In other words, you have to use up more energy than you take in. So, eat a balanced and wholesome diet in your eating phases and incorporate regular exercise into your everyday life. You don't want to do without morning exercise, but your first meal of the day is only "allowed" at noon? That's not a problem. On the contrary - training on an empty stomach has advantages.

If you stick to your stress areas, your training will be particularly effective. But you must train in your fat metabolism area. If you are on the go too intensely, the energy from burning fat is not enough. Since carbohydrates are not available, your body relies on muscle protein. This not only has a long-term negative effect on your muscle mass but also reduces performance and weakens your immune system.

The Best Intermittent Fasting Schedule? There is not any. Arrange your (non-) meal times in the way that is most comfortable for you. You can also vary the 16/8 shape. This is the most common, but alternatives such as 18/6 or 20/4 are also possible. Another option: You alternate between a fasting day and a "normal feeding day". Or you bet on "5-to-2" and fast 2 days a week and eat as usual on the remaining 5. Since intermittent fasting is not a diet, but rather a type of eating schedule, you can implement it permanently.

It is crucial that you feel good and can easily integrate your diet into your everyday life. If intermittent fasting means compulsion and stress for you, it does not make sense and will also have the opposite effect in terms of weight, because "stress hormones" promote sugar consumption and inhibit your fat burning.

CHAPTER 3

Intermittent fasting is a type of change in diet and lifestyle that, instead of drastically reducing calorie intake or skipping certain food groups, limits the times of the day you're going to eat and go fasting. In general, fasting will include bedtime and avoid eating until the end of the period. There are many schemes to implement an intermittent fasting diet, and you should pair it with exercise or calorie restriction to reduce inflammation of body tissue. That can also lead to weight loss or muscle development.

PLAN THE FAST DIET

CONSULT YOUR DOCTOR BEFORE STARTING THIS DIET

Speak to your health care provider and explain why you plan to follow a fasting diet. Tell him/her about this diet's benefits and disadvantages, and let them know about any disease you may have.

This diet will make a big impact on the day's metabolism. If you are pregnant or in poor health, do not run without consulting your doctor first.

Caution: People with type 1 diabetes who adopt an intermittent fasting diet can find it difficult to control and maintain healthy insulin levels because they never can eat food.

CHOOSE A FEEDING SCHEDULE YOU CAN MANAGE

When following this diet, you will stop eating for prolonged periods; typically, you will fast from 16 to 20 hours every 24 hours, or up to 23 hours, and in the remaining hour or the last 4 to 8 hours of the day, you will consume only full meals again. Intermittent fasting is usually a way to lose weight, and it is also an efficient way to regulate and schedule your food intake. Design and keep to a daily schedule will be critical. For example, you might slowly follow the diet by consuming only 2 meals per day. Timetable your last meal every day at the time of eating.

CHOOSE AND MAINTAIN A DAILY SCHEDULE

That allows you to eat around 2000 calories if you're a man or 1500 if you're a woman. Eat 20 to 30 calorie snacks, or less, from time to time, until the fasting ends. You can eat carrot or celery pieces; an apple quarter; 3 cherries, grapes, or raisins; 2 small cookies; or 30 g (1 oz) of chicken, fish, or similar meat. Most periodic fasting schedules are essentially the same as changing in just a few hours. You can choose from many feasible methods:

One meal period: you can fast for 23 hours a day and choose to prepare and eat a healthy meal for 1 hour a day (e.g., from 6:00 pm to 7:00 pm).

Two meal periods: eat two healthy meals a day; e.g., one at midday and one at 7:00 pm. Now fast for 17 hours after the second meal, sleep, and do not consume the "breakfast" until the fasting period ends.

Days of omission: not consuming anything on Mondays and Thursdays, and eating healthy meals for 5 days. So, you could eat the last meal of your feeding time at 8:00 p.m. on Sunday. This is known as the 5:2 diet, which consist of eating 5 days and fasting in the other 2 days.

MINIMIZE YOUR DAILY CALORIE INTAKE

When you normally eat between 2,000 and 3,000 calories a day, you can reduce the number a little during the short meals. Don't exceed 1000 or 2000 calories a day. To achieve this goal, prepare a diet that includes healthy carbohydrates, excluding white bread and noodles but some complex carbohydrates and fats.
You'll need to eat all the daily calories during 1 or 2 hours of restricted feeding.
You will find you eat fewer calories easily because you won't have time to do it during the week.

DON'T DRASTICALLY CHANGE YOUR DIET

When you follow an intermittent fasting diet, you won't have to skip any particular food class (such as carbohydrates or fats). You can eat the same food types once you start your diet as long as you follow a balanced and healthy diet and don't reach 2,000 calories per day. A diet can alter eating habits, not the food types that you consume.
A balanced diet will only include small amounts of processed foods rich in sodium and added sugars. Reflect on nutritious proteins (such as poultry and fish foods), fruits, vegetables, and moderate levels of regular carbohydrates.

FOLLOW A FAST SCHEDULE

LITTLE BY LITTLE FOLLOW THE INTERMITTENT FASTING DIET

If you're not used to fasting, your appetite, thirst, and body system may be influenced by this diet. You will follow it slowly if you extend the hours of fasting between meals or if you start avoiding food entirely on one day of the week. This will help your body to detoxify and decrease the painful symptoms (such as nausea, low blood pressure, exhaustion, or irritability) that you feel.
At the start of this diet, you can also eat light snacks during fasting times. A 100-calorie protein and a fat snack (such as nuts, cheese, etc.) won't affect how well you start and keep fasting. So, you could eat some very light snacks.
As part of this process, you will need to gradually modify your diet to reduce your consumption of processed foods such as processed meats, milk, or soda.

EAT YOUR LAST MEAL BEFORE YOU MAKE A FAST

Avoid the temptation of eating junk food, sugar, and processed foods in your last meal before fasting. Eat fresh fruits and vegetables, and plenty of protein, to maintain high levels of energy. For starters, your last meal could be a cooked chicken breast, a piece of garlic bread, and a salad made with roman lettuce, tomato, onion slices, and vinaigrette.
At the beginning of this method, some people eat compulsively but this will allow them to devote more time to food processing and less time to the "process of adaptation to fasting" of the food withdrawal period.
Eat a full meal until you start fasting. When you fill up before fasting, eating only sugar-rich foods and carbohydrates, you'll quickly feel hungry again. If you have a meal in your schedule, eat plenty of protein and fat. You might find it hard to maintain a very low intake of carbohydrates and fat, as you will always feel unhappy and hungry during the fast.

Fast During the Hours You Sleep

If you do a long fast, it will be useful not to think about the stomach's sounds. Every night you should sleep for at least 8 hours; fast for at least a couple of hours while awake or sleeping. That way, you won't feel deprived of food when you wake up because you will consume a hearty meal soon.

Upon fasting, the first meal or main course you eat will be your fasting reward. You'll feel hungry, so you should eat a full meal.

Keep Your Body Well Hydrated

You're going to fast most hours of the day if you adopt an intermittent fasting diet, but that doesn't mean you can stop drinking water. Besides, it will be important to stay hydrated during fasting to ensure your body's proper functioning. Drink calorie-free water, herbal teas, and other beverages.

This will also keep you from feeling hunger pain, as the liquids will fill the abdomen area.

Fasting and the Hormones

Fasting is known to be healthy, especially therapeutic fasting, intermittent fasting, and long-term fasting. Various ailments are alleviated; some illnesses are cured.

But what influence does a fasting period have on the hormonal balance? What happens to our hormones while we are fasting? Will fasting lead to aging faster because some nutrients may be missing?

Usually, one does not want to admit that aging is a part of our lives, but it affects every individual, with some being caught up with the aging process a little earlier, others later. At least that's the thesis.

It has become known that the reduction in the production of certain hormones begins around the age of 40 and is a major cause of aging. Regular fasting can have significant positive effects and largely reduce the signs of aging.

But what are the hormones on which, for example, 16/8 interval fasting has such a beneficial influence? Can you make general use of this knowledge? Is it possible to have a way of life where the negative influences of aging can be stopped?

Our Hormones Influence All Processes in the Body

Hormones determine our rhythm of life, whether it is growth, puberty, aging, inner balance, and even our health. In all areas of our life, hormones are involved in essential processes in the organism.

The proportion of the hormone DHEA produced in the adrenal glands begins to decline at the age of 25. Pronounced dehydroepiandrosterone, or DHEA for short, slows down the metabolism, reduces fat, and lowers blood pressure.

The two opponents are serotonin and adrenaline, which keep each other in check, are mostly known. With the stress hormone cortisol, which wants to convert everything into energy and makes sense in demanding situations, the DHEA slows down the increased energy burn and ensures a balanced energy balance.

You can visualize it like yin and yang, an image that stands for balance. If the production of DHEA drops, cortisone will likely gain the upper hand, which negatively affects the aging process.

But the sex hormones estrogen, progestin, and testosterone also decrease from around the age of 40. They are part of the tissue-maintaining and rejuvenating hormones. Other important hormones are serotonin and melatonin, the production of which also declines with age.

A list of important hormones that are involved in the aging process - or rather, it's slowing down:
- Serotonin (happiness hormone)
- Melatonin (sleep hormone)

- Estrogen (female cycle)
- Progestin (for water retention, female hormone)
- Testosterone (male sex hormone)
- Growth hormone STH (for body fat and muscle regulation)
- DHEA (slows down the metabolism)

On the other hand, adrenaline, noradrenaline, cortisol, and insulin (stress hormones) are unfavorable.

WHAT HAPPENES TO THE HORMONES DURING FASTING?

It is known that fasting has a positive effect on diseases such as rheumatism, arthritis, or osteoarthritis. This is related to an increase in the hormone cortisone administered in an artificial form in these diseases to curb the inflammation in the joints.

It is a reaction of the organism to the switch to the ketone metabolism, which initially means stress for the body. However, this diminishes as the fast continues and the cortisol level drops.

As the level of cortisol falls, so does the production of rejuvenating hormones such as DHEA and the growth hormone STH. The latter is even responsible for the fact that instead of muscle mass, fat tissue is broken down, which is very important in getting older. Because even from a distance, based on a person's silhouette, you can tell whether it is a young or older person.

Older people usually gain weight and build up fat deposits on the stomach, while at the same time losing muscle mass. This can lead to serious postural disorders and at some point, prevents you from getting up from the chair by yourself.

The sleep/happiness hormones melatonin and serotonin also boost their production to an appropriate extent during fasting. Especially in spring, the well-known springtime tiredness is quickly overcome with an internal spring cleaning through a fasting cure.

The serotonin level rises and the hormone melatonin ensures a particularly good sleep at night, which is also the cornerstone of a slowed down aging process.

THE POSITIVE EFFECTS OF FASTING ON OUR BODY AND THE HORMONE BALANCE AT A GLANCE

It is amazing how positively our body reacts to fasting in many different ways and how fasting hormones control us:

- Weight loss and the state of ketosis lower blood sugar levels and regulate insulin production.
- Lowering cholesterol and thus lowering the inflammatory parameters and strengthening the cardiovascular system.
- Strengthening the entire immune system with improved digestion and the associated defense against tumors and infections.
- Increasing the rejuvenating hormones like DHEA or STH and decreasing in the stress hormones adrenaline and cortisol.
- Increasing the well-being and a good mood thanks to the happiness hormone serotonin.
- Improvement of sleep quality through a balanced melatonin balance, resulting in increased stress resilience in everyday life.
- Improvement and balance of the necessary sex hormones, such as estrogens and testosterone also have a rejuvenating effect on men's and women's bodies and minds.

FASTING HORMONES - THE BOTTOM LINE

Regular fasting cures positively influence the body, regardless of your age or health situation.

Therapeutic fasting cures or intermittent fasting have a rejuvenating effect. But not only that, the hormonal balance is a very complex system, which can be unbalanced by stress or poor nutrition.

An annual fast is the best option here. Possible complaints and illnesses can certainly be associated with a disturbed hormonal balance, which can be brought back into balance by a regular fasting period.

It is not for nothing that many people see their younger, firmer skin, a special glow of the eyes, and shiny hair after the fast.

It is not a free ticket to eternal life. Still, fasting offers a completely natural opportunity to live happily and healthily with aging and at the same time with a balanced hormone balance, no matter what phase of life you are in.

CHAPTER 4

HOW THE BODY PRODUCES ENERGY WITH INTERMITTENT FASTING

Intermittent fasting is a very important tool for weight loss and health. It is about staying the day without eating. There are several ways to be done, starting in 12 hours up to 24 hours, 36 hours of fasting. Each one chooses the period that best suits their day, the use of 16-hour intermittent fasting being very common. However, many people are concerned about how our body produces ene
rgy with intermittent fasting. Many would still like to know how many hours our bodies start burning fat as the main fuel and how to manage it.

Burning Glucose from Food

Up to four hours after a meal, your body gets the energy to perform its functions through the glucose obtained from food.
This glucose is obtained mainly from carbohydrates present in sweet, floury, industrialized foods, pasta, and potatoes.
The best action for your health would be to get good carbohydrates from fruits and vegetables.
These foods are digested in our digestive system until they turn into glucose and are absorbed from the intestine into the blood.
When this exogenous glucose is used as an energy source, this period can be prolonged or shortened according to the control of your food regarding these types of foods.
Having a restricted carbohydrate diet, the body's period uses the glucose that comes from the diet as energy will be shorter.
If the glucose ingested at the last meal is too large, it is also stored as fat or glycogen and is not immediately used as an energy source.

Burning Glucose from Glycogen

After the period in which the body has used all the available glucose from the food and you continue on Intermittent Fasting, it starts using glycogen as an energy source.
Glycogen is a polysaccharide, formed from excess glucose from food, which works as a form of energy store in our liver and muscles.
This sugar is broken down and releases glucose to our body to be used as energy for our functions.
In this breakdown of glycogen, water molecules are released and eliminated from our body.
This leads to a loss of weight from our bodies.
However, in this initial phase, it is only a loss of water and not fat.
Glycogen has a limited supply that tends to last up to 24 to 28 hours in maintaining our metabolism.
Physical activities, lean body composition, and other hormonal factors vary this period of glycogen duration.

BURNING GLUCOSE FROM GLYCOGEN AND FAT

The burning of fat as an energy source for the body does not start only after zeroing the glycogen supply.

It starts from four hours after the last feeding when the meal's glucose is depleted as fuel.

This burning of fat through gluconeogenesis, where fat is converted to glucose, remains increasing until the peak around two days.

In this period, it is observed that up to 16 hours of fasting the use of glycogen as an energy source is greater than fat.

After this period, the inversion occurs.

With that, fat becomes the main energy source for our body.

What is found is that most tissues continue to use glucose from glycogen.

However, muscles, liver, and fat cells are already beginning to use fat as an energy source.

LOSE WEIGHT THROUGH AN INTERMITTENT FASTING DIET

Intermittent weight loss from fasting is a technique that has become popular over the past few years. It's a method of eating where you switch from feeding to fasting. You get to schedule your times of fasting and non-fasting, in which you drink only water. Although it is unnecessary to do intermittent fasting every other day to lose weight, it is advised for those who want to lose weight, at least twice a week.

With an intermittent fasting diet, you are allowed to eat anything you wish in the periods when you are not fasting. You'll stick to healthy foods if you're looking to lose weight and avoid those that will defeat the whole process purpose. During this time, it is recommended consuming carbohydrates as they help with fat metabolism. Drinking water is highly encouraged when you are fasting, as staying hydrated helps you lose weight more quickly. After all, you can go without food for days, but not without water.

Over the years, fasting has helped many people lose weight, and keep it off. There are a lot of reasons why it's one of the easiest ways to get into shape. If you cut your calories by continuing through scheduled fasting times, the body is forced to provide nutrition from its reserves, usually fat. Because weight loss means eating less than you're consuming, fasting lets you focus more on exercise than on a diet.

With intermittent fasting, you get relative freedom with what you eat. This is different from the many fad diets where you're limited to certain types of food. Although freedom is provided, you should only take what's right for you, as mentioned earlier. Include plenty of fiber in your diet, as it means that your body is fully working. You have to establish and stick to some sort of plan for intermittent fasting to lose weight to work. A present intermittent fasting diet plan is hard to follow, as it might not work into your lifestyle. Instead, set your days of fasting and non-fasting.

To get the hang of intermittent fasting and how weight loss happens in the everyday lifestyle with its definition, here is a summary of how to do it and take advantage of it.

CHOOSE THE 24 HOURS IF TECHNIQUE OR 12-HOUR WINDOW

It is possible to agree on several forms of intermittent fasting cycles, some differ from 24 hours plus eating on Tuesday at 6 pm and then taking the next meal on Wednesday at 6 pm. This fast shouldn't be marketed as such for long as it impacts the metabolic rate and deteriorates health in turn. The best option is to choose a 12-hour period, where fasting takes place for half a day, and then consume any fat or carbohydrate food beneficial to the body.

What happens when one meal is taken is that the body uses it until the next 12 hours and the calorie stored as fat is consumed and employed by the body when digested. It results in weight loss, and after a while, the desire and hunger pangs will also vanish as the body becomes used to it.

KEEP THE DIET SIMPLE AND SHORT

Weight loss through intermittent fasting occurs only when it is regularly practiced. There should be a plan for consistency that is simple and easily followed daily. Set food groups at intervals of 12 hours, and just have those. A simple balance of the groups will decide the intake of food necessary for the well-being of the body, healthy metabolism, and ultimately weight burning out unexpectedly. Calcium, sugar, carbohydrates, and fats can be found in the community. The only thing to do is manage it properly.

REDUCES STRESS ON THE BODY NEEDING TO SNACK TIME AND AGAIN

Intermittent fasting molds the body's needs in a way where regular snacking needs naturally die down. What happens is when extra meal intake and fat were stored in the body, that particular time is simply cut off from the daily routine and weight loss begins to occur with it. The stress the body takes in the production, absorption and use of the food, and extra meal in the consumption is also decreased. Instead, the same amount of energy is used to absorb the stored calories and burn it down by reducing fat on the stomach other body parts.

BLOOD SUGAR LEVELS AND ROUTINES ARE ADJUSTED APPROPRIATELY

Intermittent fasting has several benefits and one of them is healthy blood sugar levels as the body's intake decreases. Studies show that fewer cravings occur and this type of diet also regulates blood pressure, stress, and heart disease. Not only would intensive workouts be avoided and drastic diet cuts would not occur, but eating just about everything you want and still weight reduction happens in a span of a few months. Also, more healthy food and nutrient intake develops as a habit over a period, something that is tough to make when IF is not followed.

WEIGHT LOSS EXERCISES

TREAT YOURSELF TO SOME EXERCISE TIME

Regardless of how busy you are, you must exercise every day if you want to lose weight and not recover from the weight loss. Your simple act of walking to the store instead of driving can greatly impact how quickly you lose weight.

• Housework exercise: As many as you can mount the stairs, walk the dog three times a day, shake, sweep, and mop vigorously.

• Increasing your stage number: Instead of elevator and park, use the stairs from the store as far as possible. Start making a hobby involving moving a little while, though it doesn't seem proper exercise. Gardening, small projects, car work, or animal play are excellent ways to burn calories.

USE A CIRCUIT TRAINING PLAN

When you try to lose weight quickly for a particular event, you should follow a streamlined exercise routine. Most women's and fitness websites, just as personal trainers, offer similar streamlined workout routines designed to maximize weight loss and make weight loss noticeable within a few days of starting the regimen.

BE REALISTIC WHEN THINKING ABOUT WHAT KIND OF EXERCISE YOU WILL DO ONCE YOU BEGIN A NEW ROUTINE

If you are interested in losing weight and not regaining it, you will have to do more than a condensed exercise program. Starting with the activities you want to do and finding fun ways to do them is the best way to get started. Choosing an exercise you enjoy does not necessitate much additional motivation every day. Try out various exercises until you find one that you like, such as swimming, cycling, or even Zumba.

Remember that games like volleyball, tennis, and even Frisbee can help you burn calories while having fun to the fullest. Hence, exercise is a fun and social activity you should enjoy every day.

Start a Cardio Workout

The best form of fitness training is to include low and high-intensity aerobic exercises for the desired results. While combining cardiovascular training with resistance training is important for the body's overall health, cardiovascular training will help you lose weight quickly. Weight resistance training won't help you lose weight overnight but it can make your metabolism energy use more effective.

Make Your Exercise Routine Still Interesting

Variety is the key to keeping you happy and enjoying a healthier life. You run a higher risk of injuring yourself if you do the same exercises every day. You are also more likely to get bored, so finding the motivation to continue the exercise will be more difficult. If you're in the gym, change machines, participate in a gym class and add to your routine some resistance training.

Perform aerobic activities of low impact: moderate exercises involving brisk walking, cycling, aerobic machines, or swimming, burning calories, and keeping the heart healthy.

Lift a Little Weight

Resistance training and weight training are beneficial for people trying to lose weight because it builds muscles and increases metabolism. Approximately double calorie expenditure is achieved when aerobics and weight training are combined with weight loss strategies.

Choose Exercises That Require the Whole Body to Exert an Effort

Rest between each strength training session of the same muscle group for at least 24 to 48 hours and take 1 or 2 days off every week. You thereby exercise all muscle groups and at the same time burn calories with more muscles, as if you were doing several activities concurrently with the workout.

Get Enough Rest

Adequate rest will help you maintain sufficient energy all day long, making you less likely to over-eat and hurt yourself during physical activity. Sleep deprivation was associated with the inability to lose fat, so getting enough sleep can support you on the road to weight loss.

How to Fast Properly and Avoid 4 Mistakes That Will Stagnate You

Before choosing what kind of intermittent fasting to practice, you know the ERRORS that can ruin your health and stagnate in weight loss.

Women are very different from men when it comes to hormones and muscle mass, so we have to practice intermittent fasting differently. If you don't pay attention to these errors, you're going to fall into the same trap that many women are falling into. You're going to end up frustrated and wonder why it doesn't work for you or why you're feeling worse than you started.

Let's move on to the mistakes women make when carrying out intermittent fasting.

Error # 1

DO NOT GRADUALLY STORE!!! If you're not used to making long and sudden fasts for 16-24 hours, your body's going to experience a shock and your hormones are going to leave equilibrium. This can hurt your metabolism and you will end up depressed and sick rather than losing weight.

Continue introducing intermittent fasting slowly. Compress the time window you eat slowly and increase the time window you are fasting in.

For example, if you're used to dinner at 8 p.m. and breakfast at 6 a.m. the next day, then try dinner at 6 p.m. this week and have breakfast at 6 a.m. This will increase your fasting window from 10 hours to a 12-hour window. Do it for 1 week and evaluate how you feel!

If you don't experience many cravings, headaches, or any other negative symptoms, then increase your fasting hours by 1 or 2 more hours the following week.

Error # 2

DO NOT LIST YOUR SERVICE! This is one of the WORST errors that you can make. Most women choose to fast for 18 hours, and while their body screams that they are starving, they do not eat even if they feel weak because 18 hours have not gone by.

What a fatal error!

This action just causes slow metabolism and the body sticks to fat.

This is why you should always listen to your body. Follow the intermittent fasting method of intuition. Let you be driven by your body! Hear the signals your body is giving you ALL TIMES!

If when you are doing an X hour of fasting you feel weak, you have headaches, you are hungry excessively, you feel that you are going to pass out, or that you want to vomit... ALL these are symptoms you are exceeding yourself in the number of hours of fast. What are you doing and what do you need to eat?

This does not mean you will never be able to fast for X hours. It just means that your body is not yet ready for such a long fast and that you have to start with a slightly shorter fast which you will gradually increase.

Error # 3

THE SAME AS MEN OR THE SAME AS WOMEN! As a woman, finding the type of fasting that fits our lifestyle and body type best is MUST IMPORTANT. Generally speaking, what works for men does not work for women. It may not work for you what works for me! We are all different, and the speed that suits your body best may vary from your mate, neighbor, aunt, etc. So, try different schedules to see which one is best for you and which one fits with your daily activities. Try versatility.

For example, if you usually have dinner at 6 p.m. and have breakfast at 10 a.m. the next day, but today you have an event with friends where you'll have dinner until 8 p.m. You can have dinner at 8 pm and switch your lunch for midday or just fast a little shorter the next day. NOTHING IF YOU MOVE THE SCHEDULE A LITTLE LESS!

You don't have to fast every day for 16, 18, 20, or 24 hours! You can vary the hours of fasting that you do every day.

The hours of fasting that I do daily vary depend on how hungry I am or what activities I have that day. This gives me the flexibility to feel good at all times .

Error # 4

DO THE FAST OF THE KETOGENIC DIET! Do NOT fly with the ketogenic diet intermittently! It's going to be a huge shock to your skin. If you have been practicing the ketogenic diet for a while now, then you can begin to implement intermittent fasting. However, if you're a ketogenic diet beginner, let your body first adjust to this new eating style and then introduce intermittent fasting.

When you introduce these concurrently, the body will resist so many changes and try to protect itself by sticking to the food and nutrients it receives rather than using them freely.

Even I would recommend starting with the ketogenic diet first and then adding intermittent fasting after a few months of practicing the ketogenic diet.

With the ketogenic diet, you will receive far more health benefits and weight loss than with intermittent fasting. This does not mean intermittent fasting is not a fabulous tool for burning fat and health... It just means it's a more advanced tool to give our metabolism an extra boost once it's in a fat-burning mode and on the way to better health.

CHAPTER 5

INTERMITTENT FAST AND HEALTH

Studies on the potential benefits of fasting have emerged in recent years, particularly since the 2016 Nobel Prize was awarded to the Japanese Yoshinori Ohsumi medical team to discover the health benefits of the metabolic process called autophagy. It is a method by which the body is able to eliminate aberrant structures, so that altered or tumor cells, viruses, bacteria, and other structures are simply "engulfed" by lysosomes, macrophages, and other immune system-derived processes that occur mainly in periods of fasting. It has been observed that autophagy occurs in the body after approximately 12 hours of fasting due to the activation of the AMPK metabolic pathway when glucose and insulin are at low levels.

Metabolic Syndrome

Without a doubt, both metabolic syndrome and all associated processes can be improved thanks to fasting. For example:
- Blood glucose and insulin fasting.
- HDL lipoprotein boost.
- Reduced visceral fat and lower triglycerides.
- Blood pressure control.
- Blood coagulation improvement and thrombosis and cardiovascular disease prevention.
- Development of the predisposition of metabolic syndrome-associated benign and malignant tumors.

Some studies have an influence with respect to different cholesterol fractions on the positive effect of fasting so that LDL appears to decrease and HDL to increase.

Intermittent Fasting and Blood Pressure

Although there are no official trials in which increases in blood pressure have been shown in intermittent fasting, we find that patients who have been gradually decreasing calories for several days have more than apparent a drop in blood pressure. Up to 80% of subjects experience a significant drop in blood pressure from 3 or 4 days of fasting. We must bear in mind that, when a person fasts, insulin levels tend to decrease. We know insulin is pro-inflammatory; it increases sodium retention and helps to produce fluid retention in the body, which has a negative impact on blood pressure.

Fasting and Weight Loss

It should be remembered that one of the benefits of trying to limit the number of calories to 8-10 hours is that people usually end up consuming less. The studies conducted by Varady Et. Al in 2013 found that for 12 weeks the correlation between a group of people who ate food for many hours and another who practiced intermittent fasting resulted in an average reduction of 5.2 kg (10 pounds approximately) between the second of the listed groups after a few weeks. A fat reduction of 3.6 kg (7 pounds approximately) has also been observed, which is explained by the fact that there are more hours of low insulin levels when fasting, which promotes metabolic activation associated with fat loss.

Some athletes are afraid that the fasting will result in a loss of muscle mass caused by proteolysis. However, numerous studies have been conducted in which the amount of nitrogen in urea (a good indicator of proteolysis) has been tested, concluding that it does not increase until 60 hours of fasting. There should be no concern about the loss of muscle mass.

An interesting fact demonstrated by scientist is that when undergoing an obese population nucleus, they both lose the same amount of weight relative to another group that performs fasting. Those who practiced intermittent fasting, however, decreased more kilos associated with fat mass (90%) compared with fat-free mass (10%). The group which performed a continuous caloric restriction lost 75% of weight in fat mass and up to 25% of fat-free mass, which means greater muscle mass loss and appears to achieve a lower basal metabolic rate after a few weeks (as opposed to those that perform intermittent fasting).

People who make an ongoing caloric restriction have more problems with increased appetite, heart output, thyroid-level hormonal imbalances, growth hormone, glucagon, adrenaline, testosterone, etc. This does not happen, and even some parameters improve in people accustomed to fasting. We also know that, in subjects who perform fasting, levels of leptin, ghrelin or adiponectin tend to be much more regulated. This means that appetite and satiety balance are more controlled because these hormones are directly responsible for these sensations.

INFLAMMATION AND INTERMITTENT FASTING

We're stopping at people fasting in Ramadan. Modulation and enhancement of inflammation-related biomarkers (such as C-reactive protein, interline 6, or Alfa tumor necrosis factor) were observed. People who made Ramadan appeared to lower the body's levels of inflammation. We find that the activity of the AMPK enzyme pathway increases after 12 hours of fasting, consistent with autophagy and immune system regulation with reduced body inflammation.

BIORHYTHMS AND FASTING

Intermittent fasting imposes a diurnal pattern on the organism's food consumption, which makes the person adapt better to the biological cycles of day/night. The organism consumes food for 8 hours a day, and the intake will not be done during the following 16 hours. The body recognizes eating during daylight hours and the hypothalamus receives an activation that has a very positive effect on the rest of the glandular, hormonal and immunological function.

The digestive system is one of the systems that most benefit from regulating circadian rhythms, as many of its functions are closely related to these rhythms. For example, stomach emptying, blood flow at mesenteric vessel level (which must be higher during the day than at night), as well as all metabolic functions associated with the pancreas, gallbladder, or liver. This allows all digestive metabolic functions to be active during the day and slow them down at night.

Likewise, it has been shown that when food is ingested at night, the quality and duration of sleep are usually affected. At the same time, there is an impact in insulin resistance, in the release of growth hormone, and in different neurohormones linked to tissue recovery and repair.

FASTING AND BRAIN FUNCTION

Fasting has a beneficial effect on the brain's level of neuronal activity. First of all, by recomposing the organism in the day/night cycles, a very positive hormonal modulation causes the dopamine levels to be high in the morning (which allows the person to be very active). The serotonin levels will remain high at night, which will be beneficial to the rest by having the lowest levels of fasting insulin. A greater release of growth hormone and more neurotrophic factor derived from the brain are permitted at night, which makes the person more neuroplastic and can prevent much better neurodegenerative pathologies like Alzheimer's, Parkinson's or multiple sclerosis. The body releases gluconeogenesis hormones (growth hormone, glucagon, cortisol and adrenaline) throughout the day by having a lower fasting blood glucose and insulin. On the contrary, people with high glucose and insulin levels usually suffer from a slowdown in mental dullness and thinking.

FASTING AND DIGESTIVE SYSTEM

Fasting methods have been used since ancient times to treat all sorts of intestinal problems such as gastritis, esophagitis, gastroesophageal reflux, bowel irritable syndrome, dyspepsia, severe fermentation, etc. In the animal kingdom, we will find a curious fact. When there is a stagnant food bolus, they need to digest or have an issue with the stomach, animals flee to fast on solid food and drink only water. This is a physiological mechanism that allows the return to equilibrium of all intestinal functions during the hours when no work is done in the digestive system.

Levels of hydration in the stomach mucosa, the release of hydrochloric acid by the stomach, or the release of enzymes and bile acids return to normal during the 14-16 hours in which the solid intake is not made. Similarly, we know that the intestinal flora continues to stabilize during fasting. The bacterial strains are balanced, causing some pathogenic strains not to proliferate excessively (e.g., Helicobacter pylori, candida, or other forms of intestinal pathogens). I have found benefits in fasting, ulcerative colitis, digestive systems, and irritable bowel syndrome.

FASTING AND CANCER

More and more scientists are trying to help cancer patients aim to change the oncological metabolic process to traditional treatments (chemotherapy, radiotherapy, surgery). In recent years, studies have been reported in which at the time of intermittent fasting in both animals and humans the modulating effects at the stage of metabolism were observed. Several volunteers underwent a study. The medical team discovered how glucose-insulin levels and, most importantly, the IGF-1 values (which is a potential oncological marker) and other cardiovascular risk indicators were greatly improved by fasting

INTERMITTENT FAST CONFECTION

It is focused on having enough fasting hours from the last to the first intake of the next day, distributing amounts of glucose, insulin, inhibiting the mTOR's anabolic pathway, and activating the autophagic pathway of the AMPK. It has been noted that this starts to happen after 12 hours of fasting, although the ideal is to arrive between the last meal and the first intake of the next day until 14-16 hours of fasting.

The instructions to follow depend on each person's schedules and customs, but the intermittent fasting rule, in general, suggests that after getting up there must be 3-4 hours in which no food has been consumed, thereby increasing the glucose levels. Insulin and gluconeogenesis hormones (adrenaline, norepinephrine, glucagon, growth hormone, and cortisol) will be released; t4 to t3 conversion will be favored and free testosterone bioavailability will be improved in the early morning hours. This will encourage the triggering of the autophagic route at the start of the day and mobilize the accumulated fatty acids in the visceral fat adipocytes.

Upon getting up, the first intake would be 3-4 hours. Some people take the opportunity to do their first fasting training They do it with low glucose and a lot of insulin sensitivity, which encourages a high-fat energy mobilization, with high lipolysis and induced thermogenesis because glucose is very small when training starts. One hour and a half or two hours before exercise are advised to make the first intake in other situations. To extend the activation of the AMPK route, this first intake should consist of protein and fat, particularly with medium-chain triglycerides found in coconut oil. In this way, the mitochondrial activity that works very efficiently from the medium-chain triglycerides will be very high.

Following the general guidance, carbohydrate intake should be done once the first practice is completed, thus breaking the AMPK route's function and activating the MTOR route linked to insulin receptor activation and hyper expression of the body's proteins. Because of this super-compensation mechanism and improved insulin sensitivity in the previous 14-18 hours, the person can assimilate the carbohydrate much better and generate a beneficial impact through insulin, enabling him to refill better glycogen and activate the routes intended for tissue formation and recovery.

Then we're going to have several more meals before we hit about 8 hours of food intake that must contain glycaemic index carbohydrates and proteins. If a person wishes to practice intermittent fasting during the seven days of the week and there are days when he does not exercise, the ideal for health purposes and to maintain insulin levels low is to reduce the amount of carbohydrate during the rest days and increase the amount of fat to have the elevated metabolic pathway of AMPK. It should be noted that fasting would not be one of the best strategies in high-performance athletes or people who eat very high calories throughout the day or are in the process of muscle hypertrophy, because in these situations you need to consume very high calories (especially carbohydrates) to have maximum glycogen levels and may cause problems at the intestinal level. Nevertheless, to boost hormonal levels and bowel functions, high-level athletes may benefit from one or two days a week of fasting.

Intermittent fasting is a technique of weight loss that involves interposing fasting periods with feeding periods. Not only "mere mortals" use this routine: athletes also use this form to remove fats that hinder their bodies.

Thanks to its simplicity, the diet is extremely popular. The approach is simply to disrupt food consumption over a certain period.

It forces the body to use its fat "reserves" to protect the biological unit. The body begins to lose weight slowly in this cycle of eating reserves.

It seems like a simple diet to do, but if you want to practice intermittent fasting, some specifics will make a difference.

The Importance of Exercise as Lifestyle

A physically active lifestyle is comparable to youth's fountain: it is one of the secrets to living longer, healthier, and happier.

Stress, along with general well-being, can be controlled through physical activity, and this is essential for achieving and maintaining a healthy body weight and reducing the risk of chronic diseases.

Among the benefits attributable to the practice of regular physical exercise, here are the main ones:
- It reduces stress.
- It improves self-esteem, self-control, and a sense of general well-being.
- It helps you keep fit.
- It helps to strengthen bones, muscles, and joints.
- It increases muscle strength and endurance
- It allows to control the bodyweight.
- It reduces the risk of chronic diseases (vascular diseases, some cancers, type 2 diabetes mellitus).
- It improves the regulation of blood pressure in hypertensive and glycemic balance in diabetics.
- It reduces states of anxiety and depression.

Physical activity and nutrition are the two most important lifestyle variables for health. Staying active increases the amount of energy consumed, which is essential for weight control. As you age, your metabolism slows down, so you need to eat less and move more to keep your energy balance constant.

IMPLEMENTATION OF PHYSICAL ACTIVITY

Incorporating into the daily routine of a constant and moderate physical activity induces a series of physiological changes in the organism that go beyond burning calories, reducing fat, and maintaining muscle mass. In addition to promoting weight loss and improving the relationship between food and the body itself, physical activity induces a change in the body's composition and the functioning of metabolism and systems (circulatory, respiratory, etc.)

Daily physical exercise, for example, is a way to improve cardiovascular health because it acts on different fronts:
* It reduces blood pressure, favoring the control of hypertension.
* It increases the secretion of HDL cholesterol (good cholesterol), reducing the rate of blood cholesterol.
* It induces a decrease in triglyceride levels.
* It decreases the production of insulin, helping to control type 2 diabetes, favoring the assimilation of nutrients, their arrival in the cells of the different tissues, and reducing the uptake and accumulation of fat.

PHYSICAL ACTIVITY

Control of cardiovascular risk factors (hypercholesterolemia, arterial hypertension, and type 2 diabetes).
* Increased lung capacity.
* Increase in muscle strength and mass.
* Increase in aerobic capacity.
* Reduction of fat mass.

It improves the person's psychological balance by inducing a state of personal satisfaction and the control of anxiety and stress.

Finally, it is worth highlighting the last benefit of physical activity. It improves the individual's relationship with food, reduces appetite, and favors the adoption of healthy eating habits.

We have to warn that in no way the IF approach can replace a direct health care provider, nor should it be used to determine a diagnosis, or to choose a procedure in particular cases.

WHAT ARE THE BEST TYPES OF EXERCISES FOR YOU (WOMAN OVER 50)?

It is time to set the table, but the exercises from 50 should be to get a healthy body. The following exercises work several muscles in your body, as well as the buttocks and hamstrings for women over 50; create stronger legs, thinner and with more force, to lift your rear part, the quadriceps also work, since they require the knee to get resistance.

To perform the first of these exercises, stand in front of a bench or a firm chair and place your left foot firmly on top of the bench or chair. Press your left foot and push the body back until the left leg is straight; lower the body down until the right knee is flexed and repeat 10 to 15 times.

Weight balanced evenly; don't lean too far forward or too far back.

The so-called bridge exercises are not only the perfect exercise for a perfectly rounded back, but they will also help women keep their back healthy and pain-free.

DEFINE ABS FOR WOMEN

To do this great exercise called a bridge, lie down on the floor with your face up, with your knees slightly bent and with your feet flat on the floor. Raise your hips so that your body shapes will take a curved line from the shoulders to the knees. Pause in the upper position for two or three seconds, then lower your body back to the initial position. Repeat this movement 10 to 15 times; then take a short rest of five minutes maximum and repeat the number of times before recommended.

The addition of raising an arm while performing the previous exercise on the floor improves the posture and the strength of the base, which makes me feel better. It will seem more effort, but you will feel more secure. Given the situation of reducing our belly, it is important to perform the exercises constantly and linearly; it is advisable to expand the abdominal table for women progressively. Every 10 or 15 days would be correct because each time we will have the most strengthened abdominal area.

STRENGTHEN BUTTOCKS

To perform the following exercise for women over 50 to create stronger, stronger legs and buttocks, start by adopting an iron position, but bend your elbows and lean on your forearms instead of on your hands.

EXERCISE TABLE FOR THE BUTTOCKS

Your body should create a straight line to the ankles from the shoulders. Tighten your buttocks and maintain your hip position while raising your right arm forward; move your shoulder blades down and back as you raise your arms. Keep the position for 5 to 10 seconds; relax the buttocks and repeat the exercise ten to fifteen times, alternating arms.

Yoga has so many physical and mental benefits. The postures are excellent to help reduce the appearance of cellulite. Make shoulder support or put your legs above the wall for 5 minutes every night before going to bed. This will be beneficial not only for the appearance of cellulite but also to collaborate greatly with leg circulation.

EXERCISES FOR WOMEN OVER 50 YEARS TO CREATE STRONGER, THINNER, AND STRONGER LEGS

To correctly perform the following exercise after 50, you have to take it more calmly. To create stronger, more firm legs and buttocks, lie on your back and gradually lift your hips and legs off the floor, bringing your legs above your head until your toes touch the ground behind you. Place your hands behind your back and extend your legs stretching them in the air, creating a straight line from your shoulders to your ankles.

Keep your neck relaxed and your shoulder support hold, try to hold the position for at least one minute and then slowly reach the starting position, pause, rest, and then repeat the movement about ten more times, obviously with your respective breaks.

For a quick toning of the whole body, go through the movements described above and perform three sets of exercises about ten times or otherwise indicated by a medical condition; move as quickly as possible between the movements to the maximum calorie intake.

The next day, do other exercises. You can incorporate a few series of cardio intervals at the time of training your entire body; or you can do it separately over a longer period in these exercises for women over 50 years. If you want to reinforce a specific part of your body, you should focus on exercises that train those particular muscles and incorporate them into your daily regimen. To continue to be effective, you should gradually increase the number of repetitions concerning how strong the muscle gets.

AN EXERCISE ROUTINE FOR WOMEN OVER 50

Multidirectional exercises help develop coordination and control while providing toning and hardening of the quadriceps, buttocks, hamstrings, and inner thighs.

To perform the following exercise, stand with your feet together, both arms stretched over your head, palms facing foward. Take a wide step with your right foot towards the corner of the room at a 45-degree angle and diagonally, bending the right knee and reaching the lower part of your body in a forward motion on your right thigh. The back leg should be straight, with your heel lifted off the floor.

LEG AND BUTTOCK EXERCISES

If you can touch the ground, do it on both sides of your right foot, lightly with your fingers. Push with your right foot to return to the starting position. Repeat 15 times on one leg and 15 times for the other. An option to modify this exercise is not to go so low in the stride and aim to reach with your hands at the knee or the level of the shin instead.

LEG EXERCISES FOR WOMEN

As quick advice, stand again out of the position described above and focus on working out the abdominals with tight buttocks, squeezing your thighs together, and maintaining good posture.

In addition to getting thinner and stronger legs, the postures that we must adapt maintain a healthy and erect back. In addition to hardening our legs, our day to day will have a better quality of life. Now I remember what it cost to climb the stairs with a smile from ear to ear.

CHAPTER 6

HOW THE WOMAN'S BODY CHANGES

The body does not stop changing throughout our lives. Age and genetics are primarily responsible for these changes, although not the only ones. External factors such as tobacco, alcohol, poor diet, or excessive sunbathing are determinants for our health's deterioration over the decades.

In women's case, the number of hormones that we have determines the evolution of our body over the decades. Fertility is also key to understanding the changes that occur. Between the decades of the 20s and 60s, the woman undergoes a series of important changes, both hormonally and physically, as a result of menstrual cycles, pregnancies, and other derivatives of reproductive aging.

At 20 Years Old

During this decade, the woman is full of energy and performance and enjoys a baseline health status. The body adapts to our rhythm of life and we perform better physically.

Genetics is a fundamental factor that determines endogenous aging; however, everything takes its toll. As much as at 20 years the skin is full of collagen, but a weekend of excesses on the beach or smoking daily are points that accumulate against the epidermis and time. If a person with a genetic predisposition to have a thinner dermis or lighter skin, also smokes, sunbathes, and has excessive gestures, may have wrinkles in the 20s.

Creating good exercise habits while avoiding alcohol and smoking, paying attention to eating disorders and attending gynecological exams annually must be part of a woman's routine after the 20s.

As for the skin, during this decade and the third, the woman loses the brightness of adolescence and therefore must start using moisturizers, which should subsequently be rich in alpha-hydroxy acids.

During the second decade, the woman is in the fullness of her sexual development by ovarian activity. The secretion of hormones such as estrogen and progesterone play a fundamental role in the menstrual cycle and fertility.

At birth, our ovaries have a million oocytes and will no longer be produced. In each menstrual cycle, they are discarded, so as time progresses the possibility of becoming a mother decreases until menopause arrives. Between the ages of 15 and 25, the probability of becoming pregnant in each cycle is 40 percent. During this time, contraceptive treatments should be taken into account to avoid unwanted pregnancy and assist in the transmission of infectious diseases.

At 30

From the age of 30, there is a decrease in metabolism, which means that we naturally burn fewer calories per minute if we do not exercise.

The specialist Concepción de Lucas points out that if you also lead a sedentary lifestyle, with work stress, or poor diet, your physical condition can worsen.

Also, this is the decade in which many women have their first child: the average is 32 years old. The expert points out that this moment is key for women. "In this decade, muscle tone is lost and, with pregnancy, the body can undergo significant changes, with increases and decreases in weight, body volume, and muscle sagging."

It is also common to observe adult acne, which usually appears in the jaw area and that is due to excessive sensitivity of the skin of that area to hormonal changes. That can be treated with synthetic prescriptions or oral remedies, including contraceptives (not indicated for pregnant women since it can cause alteration is in the fetus), as dermatologist María Teresa Tracheole explains. This type of acne may also be due to disorders such as the polycystic ovary or the use of overly fatty cosmetics.

From the age of 30, expression wrinkles begin to appear in the areas where we are most gesturing, such as between the eyebrows or the eye area, with bags and crow's feet. The specialists recommend using moisturizers and containing active ingredients such as the alpha, as mentioned earlier, hydroxy acids, which seek to reshape the skin, vitamin C, and niacinamide.

You have to maintain good eating, exercise habits, and go to gynecological exams annually. Do health checks to monitor cholesterol, weight, visual, auditory acuity, and the early detection of diseases and pathologies.

From the age of 35, the woman's fertility decreases and it is increasingly difficult to get pregnant. Gynecologists advise not to delay motherhood beyond this age because, in addition to having to resort to assisted reproduction techniques, they add the risks of having abortions, hypertension, diabetes, and deformations or alterations in the fetus. From the age of 40, the probability of pregnancy in each cycle is 25 percenT.

At 40

During the fourth decade of our life, a series of changes in our physiognomy begin to occur. The fat that predominated in the buttocks and legs for possible breastfeeding begins to redistribute in the abdomen, increasing cardiovascular disease risk.

Also, decrease muscle mass and tone and increases sagging in arms and legs, especially if we do not exercise. The level of hormones drops and the woman is moving away from her period of greatest fertility.

The skin loses elasticity and sunspots begin to develop like antigens, which are more marked on the lighter skins. Expression wrinkles intensify, and facial volumes begin to vary. The expert recommends anti-spot lasers, botulinum toxin for expression wrinkles, and hyaluronic acid to treat the anogenital groove's wrinkles and volume loss.

Good eating habits and exercise will contribute to a better menopausal transition in the future, as Lucas warns. The specialists indicate that, from the age of 40, the tendency to suffer from hypertension and cholesterol, pathologies observed in men, rises.

Also, the intervertebral discs are compressed, and it is normal for spine pain, loss of muscle tone to increase, and osteoporosis or loss of bone mass. It is important that young women prevent their appearance by performing a diet rich in calcium and muscle strength exercises. This serves to condition the muscles, make them stronger and stronger. It also strengthens the union of muscle with a bone through tendons.

From 45-50 years old, women can begin to notice hot flashes, irritability, difficulty sleeping, vaginal dryness, decreased libido, and alterations in menstruation; "We are in premenopause," explains Esparza, who advises to see it as "a natural stage in women," which must be normalized and treated if necessary, to reduce symptoms. "We must not fear it, no methods can prevent it, simply accept it as another stage as a person and as a woman. From the age of 45, early menopause can also occur, which usually occurs between 50 and 55 yeaRS.

During the 50s, women begin to suffer from menopause, which is the absence of menstruation for more than 12 months and is due to the permanent cessation of follicular function. Its diagnosis is clinical and retrospective when 12 months have elapsed since the last period without any menstrual bleeding.

Lucas's conception clarifies that "there are no clear guidelines on how to deal with it because each woman has different experiences, but most of the changes in their bodies are related to it."

During this period, the alteration in the distribution of body fat continues. The appearance of the skin in terms of elasticity and hydration worsens; vaginal dryness and other mucous membranes that can cause pain during sexual intercourse are experienced; muscle tone decreases, and muscle damage deteriorates. Bones of the spine, joints, or osteoarthritis problems appear.

"It also increases cardiovascular risk, sleep and memory disorders influenced by the gradual loss of estrogen," explains the specialist, adding that lifestyle changes can cause several mood changes: "during this stage, it is normal to suffer more anxiety, depression and a decrease in mood."

In the fifth decade, the woman may also notice that she loses pubic and axillary hair and undergoes changes in hair and skin or increases in body weight.

Menopause causes that; between 50 and 60 years, the woman's skin experiences many alterations. "The decrease in estrogen that occurs at this time in the woman's life leads to a thinning of the skin and dehydration, which causes wrinkles to intensify and 'sagging' of structures.

You should try acclimatizing the body to the symptoms of menopause by reducing body temperature with light clothing, drinking cold drinks and exercising regularly to prevent osteoporosis. Proper nutrition, doing controlled breathing exercises, going to gynecological exams, and other medical check-ups are also tipping to keep in mind during this stage and during the sixth decade of our life.

The specialist also recalls that throughout the woman's life, the gynecologist must be present, adapting her actions to the different health and reproductive status.

At every stage of the woman, physical changes and psychological changes occur, so that the specialist must be a foothold to ask constantly. "These are vital phases that must be accepted and lived. You don't understand or doubt you have; you will have your gynecologist to solve THEM.

Process of the Change of Our Body and the State of Well-Being

Our health and well-being have taken priority in our daily lives: when we have free time, outside of work and when we are not occupied with occupations, we like to devote ourselves to activities that are healthy and fun: spending time with friends, playing sports, attending social gatherings, or participating in cultural activities, for example.

But, how do we go about attaining mental and physical well-being that will allow us to enjoy life every day and reach our full potential? We learn about new ways to promote our physical and mental health every day, but much information is still out there, and we may not have as much time as we deserve to familiarize ourselves with our health. Therefore, we are featuring a compilation of the best methods to help you feel physically and mentally hEALTHY.

Break with a Sedentary Lifestyle

It does sound a bit cliché, but our way of life is exceptionally sedentary. At times we find ourselves suffering from the stagnation that could lead to depression because we are not taking advantage of our bodies and our surroundings (or, without going too far, to procrastinate and waste our free time, making us feel that we do not give up or take advantage of the time we have been given). Getting out into the world is an excellent way to escape this vicious cycle. This simple action could mean a considerable change in our mental state, especially for those who make it happen physically (something that always produces a feeling of health that raises our mood). Make sure you spend some time outside every day. If you spend this much time exercising in the fresh air each day, you should be able to smell the difference in your skin and hair in a few weeks. Walking is one of the healthiest exercises, and it burns the same calories as running, but it requires more effort because we walk faster. Relax and clear THE MIND.

Try New Cultural Activities

This may sound like an exaggeration, but every day of our lives we have the opportunity to experience new things. It is common for travelers to participate in cultural activities that enrich their travel experience. There are activities like watching plays, attending concerts and participating in cultural fairs where one can meet and learn about other cultures, explore different cultural movements of one's own country, and discoveR NEW ONES.

Play Sports

To have a complete and healthy lifestyle, people must engage in regular exercise, maybe playing sports. There are ways to improve both mental and emotional well-being. However, getting physically fit not only occurs in training but is also a way to gain benefits in other areas of life. Conducting exercise not only loosens our bodies but also exercises them, preventing them from atrophying. Another benefit of muscle growth is that it helps our physical appearance, and that, in turn, helps individuals to have a greater sense of self-confidence.

Beyond this, sport also offers a period of a shared company in the weekly routine that greatly benefits the individual. It offers opportunities for both work and play, enhancing social interaction in a very positive way. Regardless, physically fit people can practice physical exercise alone or in their home, doing various exercise routines every day. Keep in mind that physical exercise causes endorphins to be produced, which is the same as feeling happy whILE DOING IT.

New Experiences (extreme sports)

You can also try out some new types of physical activities that can contribute to your workout routine while also discovering a new skill within yourself. An example is the aerial fabrics, which are in style now and can be practiced in a sports center or at home, and the wind tunnel, in which we can simulate what it is like to practice skydiving. We have in this line the type of sports where you take all of your adrenaline, and these are known as adrenaline sports. Also, you have sports like bungee jumping or any form of extreme sport that enables you to leave your stress behind and facE SOMETHING NEW.

Establish Routines

ROUTINES ARE THE GROUNDWORK FOR A HEALTHY LIFE AND A SATISFYING EXISTENCE. IN REALITY, THE VOLUME OF CHAOS WE EXPERIENCE HOURLY DOES NOT LEAD TO GREATER FULLNESS IN OUR LIFE. INSTEAD, IT CREATES A FLUCTUATING AND DISORDERED SYSTEM IN WHICH OUR DAILY SCHEDULE FOR HUNGER AND SLEEP BECOMES THROWN OFF. THIS CAN LEAD TO INSOMNIA (A VERY SERIOUS PROBLEM TODAY). IT MAY BE THAT A SYSTEM AIDS THINKING SYSTEMATICALLY BECAUSE IT ENCOURAGES THE STANDARDIZATION OF DAILY TASKS AND AIDS IN CREATING AN ORGANIZED AND WELL-STRUCTURED MANNER OF THINKING FOCUSED ON A PARTICULAR OBJECTIVE. BY CREATING SCHEDULES AND ROUTINES, WE CAN MAXIMIZE THE TIME THAT WE HAVE TO COMPLETE OUR WORK. THIS HELPS US ACCOMPLISH OUR DUTIES FASTER AND MAKES IT EASIER TO COPE WITH OUR STRESS.

Cultivate Hobbies and Have Habits

Our hobbies are a representation of our personality, which means exploring our hobbies is a way of learning more about ourselves. A fantastic way to commune with ourselves every day is to regularly explore new hobbies, as well as our current ones. Doing so will also help us forge new friendships, which are a key component to maintaining our OVERALL WELL-BEING.

STAY AWAY FROM BAD COMPANY AND CONSULT YOUR Concerns with a Specialist

To cultivate emotional and mental health, the most important point is to understand ourselves. To stay mentally and physically fit, we must allow our brain to recuperate after periods of stress or take advantage of help when we require it. Considering our problems with a mental health professional (like a psychologist) is a great way to help maintain our overall mental and emotional well-being; it's like having a periodic physical health check-up. Alternatively, to take a step away from corporations that use up our resources and influence our daily lives for the worse, we must leave them behind to strengthen our positivity. Indeed, it is possible to improve your physical and mental health. The suggestions listed here can help you on your path to living a full life every day.

CHAPTER 7

FOOD TO EAT AND DRINK AND WHAT YOU MUST AVOID

During fasting periods, the person can drink water, teas, and coffee without sugar, regardless of the strategy adopted.

Knowing what to eat in food windows is just as important as fasting since with the right food the body takes better advantage of fasting.

It is also recommended to have the assistance of a nutritionist to practice intermittent fasting, as this professional will be able to set up the best diet for you.

Below we list some foods that can be part of the menu of fasting practitioners.

Foods That Should Be Consumed

• Avocado: rich in healthy fats. Studies show that adding half an avocado in between can keep the body free from hunger for a few hours straight;

• Fish: are excellent sources of protein and also healthy fats. It is recommended to consume fish at least twice a week;

• Sweet potato: it is one of the best options for those who want to do intermittent fasting, as it serves as a source of healthy fibers and carbohydrates, generating a feeling of satiety. Choose the baked or roasted version;

• Eggs: they are another source of protein, just like fish. In addition to having excellent levels of protein, they are rich in many nutrients, helping to maintain muscle mass and energy during fasting;

• Nuts and chestnuts (cashew nuts, from Pará, and others): they are great options for snacks, as they are rich in calories, proteins and also in fibers, which can contribute a lot to the feeling of satiety;

• Whole grains: they are great sources of healthy carbohydrates and fiber. They can be inserted in main meals, snacks, and breaks. Studies suggest that consuming whole grains instead of refined grains optimizes metabolism and even favors weight loss;

• Probiotics: are substances that help the intestine to function well. The yogurt, the kefir, and fermented milk foods are examples of such substances;

• Cruciferous vegetables: this group of foods includes vegetables such as broccoli, cauliflower, and Brussels sprouts-all rich in fiber, a nutrient known for its ability to promote satiety for the body, in addition to contributing to intestinal health;

• Foods rich in flavonoids: A 2015 survey found that people who followed a diet rich in flavonoids decreased their BMI (body mass index) over the years.

Eat Nutrient-Balanced Meals

During feeding periods after fasting, the body must receive balanced meals in nutrients to stabilize metabolism. Each meal must consist of:

• Healthy carbohydrates (including fiber-rich foods like brown rice or sweet potatoes);

- Healthy proteins (lean meats like some chicken cuts, beef cuts, or fish);
- Many vegetables, beans or lentils, as well as a variety of vegetables;
- Essential fatty acids (fish, nuts, and seeds).

Also, it is important to know that intermittent fasting only has positive effects if the food eaten during meals in the feeding window contains a high nutritional value.

INCREASE YOUR CONSUMPTION OF WATER AND HEALTHY DRINKS

Water is essential for all metabolic processes, being necessary to reduce weight and body fat. It is recommended to consume at least 35 ml of water per kilogram of weight.

When the body is dehydrated, symptoms of fatigue, headaches, tiredness, among others, may appear.

Increase your intake of water, unsweetened teas, or coffee, which can also assist in metabolism activation, promoting a thermogenic effect.

WHAT FOODS TO AVOID

The chosen foods must be healthy, avoiding processed or fatty foods as much as possible:
- Candy;
- Industrialized cookies;
- Frozen or canned foods;
- Ready sauces;
- Whole dairy products;
- Refined cereals (including rice and white bread);
- Fried snacks;

Also, it is recommended not to use too much salt and sugar in the preparation of food.

TIPS ON HOW TO SAFELY DO INTERMITTENT FASTING

FACILITATE YOUR NEW EATING PLAN

While it can be tempting to go directly into your new eating routine (the initial excitement is real), it can be difficult and make you hungrier and more uncomfortable. It is best to start slowly, doing two to three days of intermittent fasting during the first week, and then "gradually increasing week by week".

KNOW THE DIFFERENCE BETWEEN WHEN TO EAT AND WANTING TO EAT

After hearing your stomach growl, it may seem like there is no way to go more than X hours without food. Understand this question: ask yourself whether hunger is boredom or real hunger. If you are bored, get distracted by another task.

If you are really hungry but don't feel weak or dizzy (which are signs you should stop fasting as soon as possible), have a hot mint tea, as mint is known to reduce your appetite, or drink water with lemon (don't add sugar) to help fill your stomach until your next meal.

Now, if you have been trying to do intermittent fasting for some time and still feel extreme hunger between periods, you need to think about it. You need to add more nutrient-or calorie-rich foods over the eight hours or consider that this may not be the best plan for you. The addition of healthy fats, such as nuts, peanut, avocado, coconut butter, and olive oil, as well as protein, during the feeding period, can help keep you satisfied and full longer.

Technically, intense hunger and fatigue should not occur when following the 16: 8 fasting method (perhaps the most common). But if you feel extremely dizzy, you are probably low on sugar and need to eat something.

By definition, fasting involves removing some, if not all, food. Your best bet? Make a protein-rich snack, like a few slices of turkey breast or one to two hard-boiled eggs (to help you stay in a ketogenic (fat-burning) state. You can return to fasting, of course, if you want.

Moisturize, Hydrate, and Hydrate

Even when fasting, drinking water and drinks such as coffee and tea (without milk) are not only allowed, but especially in the case of H2O, encouraged. She recommends setting reminders throughout the day and, especially during fasting periods, to absorb lots of fluids. Try to fill at least 2, if not 3, liters per day.

Break Your Fast Slowly and Steadily

After several hours without food, you can feel like a human vacuum ready to suck what's on your plate. But killing the urge in minutes is not good for your body, according to research. Instead, chew well and eat slowly to allow the digestive system to process food fully.

How to Do Intermittent Fasting: Avoid Overeating

Just because you have stopped fasting does not mean you should fill yourself with food. Eating cannot only make you bloated and uncomfortable, but it can also sabotage the weight loss goals that probably led you to intermittent fasting in the first place. Simply put: it's not necessarily how much of your plate can help you stay full longer, but what's on your plate.

Keep Balanced Meals

Having a healthy mix of proteins, fibers, healthy fats and carbohydrates can help you lose pounds and avoid extreme hunger when fasting. A good example? Grilled chicken with half a small sweet potato and sautéed spinach with garlic and olive oil.

When it comes to fruits, you want to opt for those with a low glycaemic index, which is digested, absorbed, and metabolized more slowly, causing a lower and slower increase in blood glucose. A stable blood sugar level helps prevent cravings-and therefore is critical when it comes to successfully losing weight.

Play with Different Periods

Although Hertz mainly recommends 16:8, you need to look at your overall lifestyle to see which fasting method can best fit. For example, if you wake up early, it may be best to eat during the early hours, such as 10 am to 6 pm, and fast until the next morning at 10 am. Remember: The beauty of fasting is that it is easily changeable and flexible to your schedule.

Another option is to stop fasting early and have breakfast every day to increase your strength gradually. We all naturally fast once a day-while we sleep-so maybe you do 'close the kitchen' early. For example, "close" the kitchen at 9 pm and don't eat again until breakfast at 8 am. This is an 11-hour natural fast!

How to Do Intermittent Fasting: Avoid 24-Hour Fasting

Most nutritionists do not recommend fasting for an entire day, as this can lead to weakness, hunger, and increased food consumption-therefore weight gain.

If your goal is to lose weight, considering your total calorie intake and working to reduce that weight may be more beneficial than fasting for a long time (especially if you're the type who likes to eat afterward.)

Adapt Your Exercise Routine

You can exercise if you are on a fasting diet. But you have to be aware of what types of moves you make and when. If you choose to exercise on a fast, it is preferable to do it early in the morning, when you have more energy.

Nevertheless, while you are fasting, you are not feeding your muscles properly. So, you are more likely to get hurt. Consider lower impact exercises, such as yoga or steady-state cardio, on fasting mornings, and do HIIT class after eating.

Keep Control

Believe it or not, keeping a food diary can help you with your fasting diet. Actively write down details such as emotions and symptoms (level of hunger, weakness, etc.) that arise during intermittent fasting. This can help you assess your progress. You can also write down any trigger points that make fasting more difficult, such as drinking the night before.

Listen to Your Body

This is essential! Maintain awareness of dizziness, fatigue, irritability, headache, anxiety, and difficulty concentrating. When you have any of these situations, break your fast. This confirms that the body is in starvation mode and requires nourishment. And if you begin to feel cold, it is a sign to end the fast.

Additionally, be patient. While fasting, you may feel hungrier and weaker than usual. It is okay to have these feelings for up to a week. You should abandon the diet if these difficulties last longer and if you experience similar symptoms. Do not get sick!

CHAPTER 8

WHAT IS THE OMAD DIET

OMAD stands for "one meal a day" It is a form of intermittent fasting. This menu helps you prepare OMAD safely and effectively, with enough calories and protein, to help you reach your weight loss and low-carb goals. The OMAD diet is the longest form of a limited-time window diet, equivalent to a 23: 1 fast (23 hours of fasting and ability to eat in a 1-hour time window). In its purest form, the OMAD diet does not impose a specific caloric restriction or macronutrient composition. As such, we recommend continuing the healthy low-carb diet during that meal.

Is OMAD Good for Weight Loss?

When the body is in a fasting state, it uses fat reserves as fuel for energy. This leads to the breakdown and utilization of fat, which helps in maintaining lifestyle-related disorders. It also reduces inflammation levels and increases growth hormone (HGH) levels that help burn fat.

Consumption of fibrous fruits and vegetables leads to less absorption of sugar and fat in the body. Fiber also improves digestion and relieves constipation. All of these characteristics lead collectively to weight reduction.

Advantages of the OMAD Diet:

• OMAD diet leads to weight loss: Intermittent fasting and only 1 meal per day reduce caloric intake thus promoting weight loss.

• Useful in type II diabetes: Intake of fiber-rich foods with low glycemic index controls blood sugar spikes. Weight reduction also helps reduce hyperinsulinemia.

• Heart-friendly: Reduces visceral fat and improves heart function.

• Feeling light: Intermittent fasting reduces fat deposits in the body, making you more active and less fatigued.

• Assistant for self-control: The OMAD diet inculcates the habit of selecting nutritious foods. Consciously, with practice, you will overcome your cravings and overeating.

Many of those who eat an OMAD model tend to do so just for the ease of preparing food and eating once a day. This can be especially helpful for those who travel frequently, those on shifts at work, and those with busy, hectic schedules.

Think about how much time you spend shopping, planning, and preparing meals. (And let's not even talk about dirty dishes). If there are three meals a day, how much time could you save by cutting out two-thirds?

Some people see the OMAD diet as an "easy" way to reduce calorie intake. When eating is only allowed in a 30-60 minutes time period, it becomes physically difficult to exceed your daily calorie requirements.

OMAD Diet Side Effects:

• Overeating or bingeing: When you start with OMAD, fasting for 23 hours may cause you to choose unhealthy food options. You get uncontrollable cravings for junk food and desserts. This gets better with time. As your body begins to accept the routine.

- Hypoglycemia: There is always a risk of a lack of energy. In severe cases, the person may go dark. Other symptoms include constant hunger, fatigue, shaking, inability to concentrate, and irritability. This also improves with time.
- Consistency: Calorie restriction will initially cause weight loss. But it is difficult to stick to this routine on a permanent basis. So, this may lead to weight recycling.
- Physical and Psychological Symptoms: Intermittent fasting increases stress on the body leading to anxiety-related disorders like nausea and mouth ulcers. Acidity can become a problem if your other lifestyle traits are not correct. For instance, improper sleep and OMAD in combination can lead to acidity and reflux together.
- Sleep Disorder: Intermittent fasting and calorie restriction could affect the central nervous system. This may affect the clarity, focus, and rhythm of sleep.
- Difficult to follow: It takes willpower and fortitude to stick to this diet pattern.

OMAD is definitely not a good option for those who lack motivation and cannot resist temptation.

Foods to Include in the OMAD Diet and to Avoid:

You Can Include

- Vegetables: Green leafy vegetables, carrot, broccoli, cabbage, cauliflower, red beet, lettuce, bell peppers, sweet potatoes, and squash.
- Fruits: Apple, banana, orange, grapefruit, grapes, cucumber, tomato, peach, plum, lemon, lime, pineapple, and berries.
- Animal protein: White meat such as chicken, lean meat, fish, and eggs.
- Vegetable proteins: Legumes, dal, mushrooms, soybeans, tofu, nuts, and seeds.
- Milk and its products: Whole milk, curds, cheese, buttermilk, and paneer.
- Whole grains: Brown rice, black rice, cracked wheat, millet, quinoa, and barley.
- Fats and oils: Omega-3-rich olive oil, MUFA-rich rice bran oil, sunflower butter, peanut butter, coconut oil, and almond butter.
- Nuts and Seeds: MUFA- and PUFA-rich nuts such as almonds, walnuts, pistachios, sunflower seeds, pumpkin seeds, and melon seeds.
- Herbs and Spices: Mint, fennel, thyme, oregano, garlic, ginger, onion, coriander, cumin, turmeric, pepper, cardamom, and cloves.
- Beverages: Zero-calorie beverages such as water, homemade salted lemonade, green tea, black tea, or sugar-free black coffee.

You Cannot Include

- Fruits Consume: Grapes, Jackfruit, Mango, Chikoo, Sitaphal and Pineapple in very small amounts.
- Canned foods: Canned meats, pineapples, cherries, jams, jellies or olives as it contains many preservatives, sugar, and salt.
- Milk and its products: Low-fat milk and products, flavored yogurt and cream cheese.
- Grains: with a high glycemic index such as rice and refined flour as they could lead to weight gain.
- Nuts and seeds: Limit consumption of cashews as it could also lead to weight gain.
- Fats and oils: Trans fats containing margarine, lard, vegetable oil, butter, and mayonnaise to prevent heart disease.
- Beverages: Packaged fruit and vegetable juices, carbonated drinks and energy drinks as they contain simple sugars that lead to weight gain.

Tips of What to Do and Not to Do During the OMAD Diet

Who Shouldn't Follow the OMAD Diet?
- Diabetics on insulin.
- People with severe kidney or liver disease.
- Pregnant and lactating women.
- People who suffer from hyperacidity

Simple Tips for Following the OMAD Diet for Weight Loss:
- Keep yourself sufficiently hydrated.
- Start by following the pattern for 1-2 days a week.
- Gradually increase the number of days until you feel comfortable.
- You can choose the mealtime according to your convenience.
- It is important to eat at the same time every day.
- You can consume 3-4 cups of zero-calorie green tea or spiced teas during the fasting phase.
- Consume an egg or 1 serving of nuts before working out.
- Drink coconut water after your workout to replace electrolytes.
- Get at least 7 to 8 hours of sleep.
- Avoid junk foods and fruit juices.

To Finish about OMAD
The OMAD diet is effective in weight loss and prevents weight regain. But every individual will react differently to this program. It will only work wonders if you choose a healthy lifestyle. Always consult a qualified professional before trying anything new. The best path to a sustainable life is through a healthy and balanced diet, regular exercise, and a healthy lifestyle.

The Weekly Plan of the OMAD Diet
This menu helps you do OMAD safely and effectively, with enough calories and protein, to help you achieve your weight loss and low-carb goals. This plan is recommended to be used for a defined period, as it involves one meal per day (lunch or dinner). It is simple and drama-free. Plus, you'll enjoy delicious and nutritious meals. Of course, be sure to drink plenty of water (you can also have black coffee and tea). And eat enough salt to minimize side effects like headaches.

EASY KETO BACON AND EGGS DISH

Monday Meal

5 + 10 m | beginner

Don't be shy and enjoy this classic keto breakfast for lunch or dinner. We have added walnuts and peppers to make it crisp. Why complicate things?

Ingredients:

- 70 g (2.46 oz.)smoked bacon
- 2 eggs
- 1 (200 g/7.05 oz.) avocados
- 30 ml walnuts
- ½ (70 g/2.46 oz.) green bell peppers
- Salt and ground black pepper
- ½ tbsp. fresh chives, finely chopped (optional)

At your service:

60 ml arugula
½ tbsp. olive oil

Instructions:

- The steps to follow are written for 1 serving. Take this into account if you are preparing more servings.
- Fry the bacon in butter over medium heat until crispy.
- Remove from the pan and keep warm. Leave the accumulated fat in the pan. Lower the heat to medium-low and fry the eggs in the same skillet.
- Place the bacon, eggs, avocado, walnuts, bell pepper and arugula on a plate.
- Pour the remaining bacon fat over the eggs. Season to taste.

Low carb ketogenic (kcal: 937 - We do not recommend counting calories.)

Per portion:
Net carbs: 4% (9 g)
Fiber: 16 g
Fat: 78% (78 g)
Protein: 19% (42 g)

THE CLASSIC KETO CHEESEBURGER

Tuesday Meal

20 + 15 m | Medium difficulty

Cheeseburgers ... Can there be a better entree for a keto feast? They taste good and fill you up, but they are made effortlessly! And you don't need to put them on bread to dress them with delicious Mexican sauce!

Sauce Ingredients :

- ½ (55 g/1.94 oz.) tomatoes
- ½ (7.5 g/0.26 oz.) chives
- ¼ (50g/1.76 oz.) avocados
- ¼ tbsp. olive oil
- ½ tbsp. chopped fresh cilantro
- Salt to taste

Burger Ingredients:

- 170 g (6 oz.) ground beef (minced meat)
- 60 ml (30 g/1.05 oz.) grated cheddar cheese, divided into two parts
- ½ tsp. garlic powder
- ½ tsp. onion powder
- ½ tsp. Spanish paprika
- ½ tsp. finely chopped fresh oregano
- ½ tbsp. butter, for frying

Toppings:

- 35 g (1.23 oz.) romaine lettuce
- 30 ml mayonnaise
- 35 g (1.23 oz.) cooked smoked bacon, crumbled
- 1 tbsp. chopped pickled jalapeños
- 18 g (0.63 oz.) pickled gherkins, sliced
- 1 tbsp. Dijon mustard

Instructions:

- The steps to follow are written for 1 serving. Take this into account if you are preparing more servings.
- Chop the sauce ingredients and stir well in a small bowl. Reserve.
- Mix the seasonings and half of the cheese with the ground beef.
- Assemble four hamburgers and fry them in a pan or on a grill if you prefer. Add the remaining cheese on top towards the end.
- Serve on lettuce leaves with pickles and mustard. On top, place the bacon. And don't forget about the homemade Mexican salsa!

Low carb ketogenic (kcal: 1007 - We do not recommend counting calories.)

Per portion:
Net carbs: 3% (8 g)
Fiber: 7 g
Fat: 75% (82 g)
Protein: 22% (55 g)

CARB FAT PROTEIN

KETO TUNA DISH
Wednesday Meal

5 + 10 m | beginner

Real food on a plate. Tuna, eggs, spinach, avocado, mayonnaise, and lemon. Because a keto meal doesn't have to be complicated.

Ingredients:

- 2 eggs
- 28 g (0.98 oz.) spinach sprouts
- 140 g (4.93 oz.) tuna in olive oil
- ½ (100 g /3.52 oz.) avocados
- 60 ml mayonnaise
- 1/8 lemons (optional)
- salt - pepper to taste

Instructions:

- The steps to follow are written for 1 serving. Take this into account if you are preparing more servings.
- Start by cooking the eggs. Add them carefully to boiling water and cook them for 4-8 minutes, depending on whether you like them poached or hard.
- Chill the eggs in ice water for 1-2 minutes when done; this will make it easier to peel them off.
- Place the eggs, spinach, tuna and avocado on a plate. Serve with a good dollop of mayonnaise and a lemon wedge if you feel like it. Season to taste.

Low carb ketogenic (kcal: 930 - We do not recommend counting calories.)

Per portion:
Net carbs: 1% (3 g)
Fiber: 7 g
Fat: 76% (76 g)
Protein: 23% (52 g)

CARB FAT PROTEIN

KETO ITALIAN CHICKEN WITH CABBAGE PASTA

Thursday Meal

15 + 30 m | medium difficulty

A simple and creamy dinner. Chicken, Parmesan cheese, and the tangy touch of sun-dried tomatoes. It serves you as a normal weeknight dinner or for a weekend with friends. Serve alongside butter-fried cabbage strips instead of pasta. One more success of the keto kitchen!

Ingredients:

- ½ tbsp. butter for frying
- 170 g (5.99 0z.) boneless chicken drumsticks, sliced
- 15 ml dried tomatoes in oil, finely chopped
- (35 g/1.23 oz.) cherry tomatoes cut into four pieces
- ¼ garlic cloves, finely minced
- 60 ml cream (or cream) to whip
- 75 ml (25 g/2.64 oz.) grated Parmesan cheese
- 60 ml spinach sprouts
- salt and pepper

Cabbage paste:

- 80 g (2.82 oz.) shredded white cabbage
- ½ tbsp. butter for frying salt or pepper

Instructions:
- The steps to follow are written for 1 serving. Take this into account if you are preparing more servings.
- Heat the butter in a skillet over medium heat. Fry the chicken for a couple of minutes. In this instance it is not necessary to cook it completely, since then it will continue cooking with the next ingredients. Salt and pepper.
- Add the two types of tomatoes to the pan, along with the garlic.
- Add the whipping cream. Let it boil over medium heat for about 5 minutes.
- Add the grated Parmesan cheese and simmer for another 10 minutes. Season to taste.
- Meanwhile, melt the butter over medium heat in a large skillet. Add the cabbage and fry until tender. Season to taste.
- Spread the cabbage on serving plates. Add the spinach to the pan with the creamy chicken and stir. Finally, pour the chicken along with the creamy sauce on top of the cabbage.

Tips:
- Chicken Parmesan goes great with cauliflower rice. If you want to discover more of our garnishes, here they are all.
- You can substitute the spinach for chopped kale (without the stems).

Moderate low-Carb (kcal: 653 - We do not recommend counting calories.)

Per portion
Net carbs: 5% (8g)
Fiber: 3 g
Protein: 29%(46g)
Fat: 66% (48g)

Friday Meal

15 + 30 m | Moderate

You can add all your favorite toppings to this crispy, keto, cheese-laden pizza crust that is really going to nourish and fill you up. Bon Appetite!

Ingredients base:

- 180 ml (85 g/2.99 oz.) grated mozzarella cheese
- 90 ml (45 g/1.58 oz.) almond flour 1 tbsp. cream cheese
- ½ tsp. white wine vinegar
- ½ egg
- ¼ tsp. salt
- Olive oil to grease the hands

Ingredients on the base:

- 110 g (3.88 oz.) Italian sausages
- ½ tbsp. butter
- 60 ml tomato sauce without sugar
- ¼ tsp. dried oregano
- 180 ml (85 g/2.99 oz.) mozzarella cheese

Instructions:

- Instructions are for 1 serving. Modify them as needed
- Preheat the oven to 200 ° C (400 ° F).
- Heat the mozzarella and cream cheese in a small nonstick pot over medium heat or in a bowl in the microwave.
- Mix until the mozzarella and cream cheese are melted and incorporated. Add the other ingredients and mix well.
- Moisten your hands with olive oil and flatten the dough on parchment paper to form a circle about 20 cm (8 inches) in diameter. You can also use a rolling pin to flatten the dough between two sheets of parchment paper.
- Remove the top sheet of parchment paper (if you used it). Prick the dough with a fork (all over the surface) and bake for 10-12 minutes until golden brown. Take out of the oven.
- While the dough is baking, sauté the ground sausage in olive oil or butter.
- Spread a thin layer of tomato sauce over the dough. Top with the pork and plenty of cheese. Bake for 10-15 more or until cheese has melted.
- Sprinkle oregano on top and serve with a green salad.

Advice!

Bake additional batter and freeze for a quick and easy dinner. Or, use the extra batter to make a Rosemary Garlic Focaccia Bread-just sprinkle garlic butter on top and bake for another couple of minutes.

Low carb ketogenic (kcal: 1235 - We do not recommend counting calories.)

Half a pizza:
Net carbs: 4% (13 g)
Fiber: 1 g
Fat: 74% (100 g)
Protein: 22% (66 g)

KETO CHICKEN WINGS WITH CREAMY BROCCOLI

Saturday Meal

10 + 45 m | Easy

With this simple dish, you will win over the whole world! These tender chicken wings taste like glory. Combined with the creamy broccoli they are great for weeknight dinner.

Ingredients Grilled chicken wings:

- 325 g (11.46 oz.) chicken wings
- 1/8 orange, juice and zest
- 15 ml olive oil
- ½ tsp. powdered ginger
- ¼ tsp. salt
- 1/10 tsp. cayenne pepper

Creamy broccoli:

- 180 g broccoli
- 60 ml mayonnaise
- 15 ml (0.6 g) chopped fresh dill
- Salt and pepper to taste

Instructions:

- Instructions are for 1 serving. Modify them as needed.
- Preheat the oven to 200 °C (400 °F).

- Mix the orange juice and zest with the oil and spices in a small bowl. Place the chicken wings in a plastic bag and add the marinade.
- Shake the bag well so that the wings are well bathed in the mixture. Let marinate for at least 5 minutes. If possible, allow a little more time.
- Arrange the wings in a single layer on a greased roasting pan.
- Bake on a wire rack in the middle of the oven for about 45 minutes or until the wings are golden brown and well done.
- Meanwhile, cut the broccoli into small florets and boil in salted water for a couple of minutes. They should only soften a bit, without losing their shape or color.
- Strain the broccoli and let some of the steam evaporate. Mix with the mayonnaise and dill. Season to taste.
- Serve the broccoli along with the roasted wings.

Advice!
You can substitute broccoli for small florets of cauliflower or Brussels sprouts. If you have an outdoor grill, you can also use it to cook your wings.

Low carb ketogenic (kcal: 1216 - We do not recommend counting calories.)

Per portion:
Net Carbs: 3%(9g)
Fiber: 5 g
Fat: 75% (99 g)
Protein: 22%(65 g)

22% 3% 75% ■ CARB ■ FAT ■ PROTEIN

KETO HERB BUTTER CHEESE STEAK ROULADES

Sunday Meal

10 + 20 m | Moderate

This is quite a keto delicacy. Tasty meat stuffed with cheese and served over leeks and mushrooms. A marvel for any night. And don't forget the herb butter, it adds a lot of aromas.

Ingredients:
- ½ leek
- 110 g (3.88 oz.) mushrooms
- Two thin steaks
- ½ tbsp. olive oil
- Salt and pepper
- 21 g /0.74 oz.(45 ml) cheddar cheese or gruyere cheese
- Two chopsticks
- ½ tbsp. butter for frying
- 35 g (1.23 oz.) butter with herbs

Instructions:
- The steps to follow are written for 1 serving. Take this into account if you are preparing more servings.
- Trim and rinse the leeks. Cut into wide slices, using the white and green parts. Cut the mushrooms into pieces.
- Fry the mushrooms and leeks in olive oil until they take on a good color. Season to taste. Place in a bowl and cover to keep everything warm.
- Place the thin steaks on a large cutting board. Season to taste. Place a stick of cheese on each steak and roll. Close with a toothpick.
- Sauté the roulades over medium heat for 10-15 minutes and reduce heat towards the end.
- Pour the juices over the leeks and mushrooms. Serve the roulades with herb butter and the fried vegetables. Don't forget to remove the toothpick before serving!

Advice!
You can also add a pinch of chili flakes to give the leeks a spicy touch.

Low carb ketogenic (kcal: 726 - We do not recommend counting calories.)

Per portion:
Net Carbs:3%(5g)
Fiber: 2 g
Fat: 73% (59 g)
Protein: 24%(44 g)

3% 73% ■ CARB ■ FAT ■ PROTEIN

First of all, it is impossible to know exactly how many calories you will get from a specific food, much less to know precisely what the body will do with those calories. It is much more important to choose foods that promote the release of hormones that reduce hunger, that help us stay full, and that make it easier to achieve a healthy weight.

We should focus on authentic foods that contain good quality protein, healthy fats, and nutrient-rich fibrous carbohydrates, especially vegetables that grow on the surface.

If you're having a hard time losing weight, refrain from high-calorie, rewarding foods-it's easy to lose control, even if they're low in carbs. Some classic examples are cheese and nuts.

Instead of counting calories, make all calories count: eat low-carb, nutritious, and balanced foods.

CHAPTER 9

There are certain times of the day, of the month, or the year in which those cravings to eat anything attack us. It can be between lunch and dinner, during the menstrual period, or when it is cold. Hunger attacks appear at any time, as they are caused by different factors, such as anxiety, boredom, or hormonal changes, among others. In general, you tend to eat processed foods, high in calories or high in sugar. When we eat food with a high glycemic index, the blood sugar level rises more than normal. To counteract it, the pancreas produces insulin and, as a consequence, glucose drops and we are hungry again.

When the cause is related to anxiety, it can be difficult to control. Therefore, it is advisable to go to a professional to study the case individually and recommend the appropriate treatment.

TIPS TO PREVENT HUNGER ATTACKS
DRINK LOTS OF FLUIDS

To avoid overeating, drink water before meals. The intake of liquid produces a feeling of satiety. That is why if you drink water, juices, or infusions before eating or when you feel like having a snack between meals, you will reduce the amount of food you eat and, consequently, the calories.

It is also a good idea to have a homemade broth as a first course, as it calms the appetite and avoids eating large quantities of the next dish.

CONTROL YOUR SUGAR LEVELS

If you suffer a glucose drop your appetite will skyrocket. Avoid it by eating frequently and keeping your blood glucose levels stable.

EAT WHOLE GRAINS FOR BREAKFAST

Breakfast is the most important meal and is fundamental to not feel hungry mid-morning.

Add whole grains, cookies, and fruit to your breakfasts. This will help the digestive system to function in optimal conditions.

HEAT THE FOOD

It is true that if it is not cold you do not feel like eating hot food, but it should be done, even if it is warm dishes. The reason is that studies show that hot foods send more signals of satiety to the brain than cold ones. If you heat a dish you were going to consume cold, you will contribute to making you feel fuller and, therefore, you will eat less.

DRIVE AWAY THE TEMPTATIONS

This is very effective advice because looking at food at all hours can unbalance your appetite.

Place chips, candy, and whatever tempts you to snack between meals in kitchen cabinets or opaque boxes. Instead, expose other lighter healthier foods like a platter full of fruit, grains, or vegetables.

Eat Slowly and Chew Well

The feeling of fullness occurs 20 minutes after starting to eat. If you chew quickly and, in a hurry, you can eat up to two or three times more than you really need. So it is recommended, eat slowly and chew between 20 or 30 times each bite.

In this way, you will also enjoy food more, you will feel the flavors and textures on your palate, and you will avoid acidity.

Use Small Plates to Eat

According to a study from the University of Utah, there is a lag between when a person has eaten enough and when their stomach feels full. To determine the latter, the brain fixes on external elements and receives the signal to have eaten more if the plate is left empty.

For this reason, use dessert plates to 'trick' the brain into feeling full faster.

Avoid Stress

When we have anxiety or stress, the brain stimulates the adrenal glands. These glands release cortisol, a hormone that increases motivation, including the urge to eat. Therefore, this leads you to eat more caloric foods without measure, even if you are already satiated.

To avoid reaching this situation, you must follow a balanced diet rich in foods containing vitamin B6, folic acid, and tryptophan. These nutrients promote the production of serotonin, a neurotransmitter known as the 'happiness hormone', which is involved in the proper functioning of the nervous system and also regulates appetite.

Nuts, eggs, meats, oily fish, green leafy vegetables, or bananas contain these nutrients.

Treat Yourself

Do not completely eliminate desserts from the diet because this will generate more anxiety and desire to eat. Treat yourself on time and as healthy as possible, such as an ounce or two of dark chocolate.

Sleep Well

If you sleep fewer hours than recommended, throughout the day you will be hungrier and you will crave more caloric foods (especially sweets). It is a response of the body to compensate for the energy that has not been recovered at night, so avoid it by sleeping 8 hours a day.

Finally, it must be remembered that in case of anxiety you should go to the doctor to tell you which is the most appropriate treatment for you, be it dietary or psychological.

Tips to Fill Up Earlier

We can start each of the main meals (lunch and dinner) with a hearty salad to reduce hunger.

It is better to opt for dishes with more consistency, that is, they require more chewing. For example, vegetables raw instead of cooked. Thus, you will be sitting at the table for longer and eating more slowly.

It is convenient to savor each bite well and chew more times. The brain knows when the stomach is full 20 minutes after you finish eating. Also, we will enjoy the food more; we will feel the flavors and textures on your palate and we will avoid reflux or acidity.

- Cut down on portions. The trick is not to stop eating certain foods, but to do so in small amounts. It is best to eat everything, but as a dessert plate, a good way to gradually reduce the amounts. Also, if you chew well and eat slowly you will increase the feeling of satiety and you will not be left hungry.
- Eat protein for breakfast. Not only are they essential for maintaining good muscle health, but they also have a satiating effect that will help control the urge to eat. Eating eggs or sausages for breakfast requires more energy to digest them and, therefore, more calories are burned, which keeps the metabolism active throughout the day.
- Join the real food. It is essential to eliminate refined flours, ultra-processed foods, soft drinks, and sugars from the diet, replacing them with others rich in nutrients. Choose products that are not packaged and, if you do, look carefully at the ingredients on the label to avoid additives and control the amount of salt and fat.
- Cut out sugar. It provides calories without nutritional contribution and its high intake is directly linked to weight gain, among other diseases. If you are a chronic sweet tooth, look for products that do not have sugar or fat.
- Drink two liters of water daily. It is very important to regulate weight because it helps eliminate toxins and purify the body and increases energy expenditure thanks to a mechanism known as thermogenesis, which speeds up metabolism. Also, it has a satiating effect since drinking water before meals makes us feel fuller. Drink at least a liter and a half and, if it costs you, add flavor with some fruit or opt for warm infusions.

CHAPTER 10

SUPPLEMENTS AND INTERMITTENT FASTING

Intermittent fasting consists of alternating periods of feeding with others of fasting. Depending on the hours that we extend the time without eating, we will carry out one type of fast. The most common are 10 or 12 hours of fasting but it can also be extended to 24 hours.

According to different research, with 10 to 16 hours of fasting, the body already begins to notice the benefits of this resource, converting its fat reserves into energy and releasing ketones into the bloodstream.

It is important to include supplements that do not interfere with it or even help us make it more bearable during our fasting stage. These supplements can help us improve energy, reduce hunger and even give us a feeling of general well-being.

After getting to know the different intermittent fasting protocols and knowing how this diet can affect your body and mind, learn how to potentiate its effects through supplements. But first, an important warning: for your weight loss to be even more effective, do your workouts immediately before breaking your fast, so that right after the exercises you can eat. This strategy optimizes the recovery and synthesis of proteins and replenishes their energies.

Top Supplements for Intermittent Fasting

BCAA's

When you are in a fasted state, you cannot have anything with calories. This can be very difficult when you are having a bad day and feeling hungry. It can also cause unnecessary muscle breakdown to support the body. Enter BCAAs-the savior of both problems. Branched Chain Amino Acids will have 0 calories and will prevent muscle breakdown when consumed. They will help fill you up so you can get to your food window.

BCAAs include leucine, and since it suppresses muscle breakdown, a BCAA supplement helps preserve muscle while you train in a fasted state.

Why not eat protein instead, you ask? Because food will increase your insulin levels and you will no longer be fasting. Whey protein is more insulinogenic than white bread.

BCAAs, on the other hand, have less of an impact on insulin levels than food, allowing you to fast while you train. That is why many people "in the know" supplement with them before fasting exercise.

Fat Burner

Most people who use IF choose to do so to lose weight. Do you want to amplify this process and keep your body energized? Enter a fat burner. This will help keep your mood and energy levels up while supporting MORE fat loss.

Yohimbine HCL (please ask for doctor's approval before taking it) is a strong compound that can assist with fat loss while on a fasting schedule. It is a stimulant that helps increase adrenaline and dopamine levels in the body; and this can cause an increase in alertness and feelings of well-being.

Up to 0.2 mg/kg of body weight is recommended. That means a 150 lb. person (divided by 2.2 to get kg) weighs 68kg and would work up to a dose of 14mg Yohimbine HCl or five capsules of Nutra BIO Yohimbine HCl a day.

Supplementation is most effective between meals or short-term fasting (empty stomach), you can divide the dose into 1 to 4 doses per day.

Example of other burners that you can use: Thermofield from Nutra BIO, is a complete fat burner since it also helps you control your hunger, increases energy, helps you with fatigue, and helps keep sugar levels stable. It's a simple formula, but as effective as Lipov 6 Black Ultra Concentrate.

MASS GAINERS (FOR BUILDING MUSCLE)

It becomes difficult to maintain a caloric surplus when you are on intermittent fasting. The window's purpose is to keep calories low and maximize nutrient absorption. To maximize your gains, you must consume enough calories. For a delicious, protein-rich mass gainer, look no further. Add it between meals and you will get an extra 300-900 calories for muscle-building. We suggest you take these supplements only if you do physical activity.

PRE-WORKOUT

If you DO and you exercise in the morning, you NEED some pre. You will need that kick in the gym since you are fasting. You just have to be careful and find a pre-workout that has 0 calories.

A suitable pre-workout fasting supplement will contain (at a minimum) caffeine and beta-alanine with minimal or no sugar. May also contain coralline, L-arginine, and creatine monohydrate.

These ingredients work together to increase muscular endurance, muscle power, focus, blood flow, and performance.

MULTI-VITAMIN

It is challenging to get three meals into your window to eat. Restricting caloric intake has a similar effect as restricting meals. Missing out on essential nutrients or vitamins for muscle building is possible. Intermittent fasting and daily multivitamins are mutually beneficial.

VITAMIN D

While prolonged fasting poses an increased risk of Vitamin D deficiency, it is still something intermittent fasting should pay attention to. Vitamin D is essential for immune health and it also helps the body absorb other essential nutrients like magnesium.

ELECTROLYTES

An important group of nutrients lost during long, intermittent fasts are electrolytes. When you are in a fasted state, ketone levels in your body increase, causing insulin levels to drop and essential nutrients are removed from the body. Although the numerous roles played by electrolytes, including sodium, magnesium, chloride, phosphate, potassium, calcium, and bicarbonate, are varied, they are essential for the nervous and muscular systems. A proper balance of electrolytes is also critical for ketogenesis, the process of converting fat into energy.

Depending on the type (s) of electrolytes missing, the symptoms of electrolyte deficiency can vary. These symptoms include:

- Nausea
- Fatigue

- Threw up
- Muscle weakness/spasms
- Headaches
- Irregular heartbeat

The possibility of low electrolyte symptoms causing a significant problem for those on a fast should be considered. An electrolyte imbalance and its symptoms can be avoided by ensuring you are giving your body enough of these essential nutrients while you are fasting.

Increasing the potassium, sodium, and magnesium levels are the most important electrolytes to supplement while on an intermittent fasting regimen. Without these three elements, which are easy to eliminate when fasting, our bodies would be deficient in the substances that maintain the proper balance of fluids and keep our blood pressure stable.

Magnesium and probiotics

Magnesium is a mineral found in various foods such as seeds, peanuts, and milk. It performs various functions in the body, such as regulating the functioning of nerves and muscles and helping to control blood sugar.

The daily recommendation for magnesium consumption is usually easily achieved when eating a balanced and varied diet, but in some cases, it may be necessary to use supplements, which must be prescribed by the doctor or nutritionist.

WHAT IS MAGNESIUM FOR?

Magnesium performs functions in the body such as:
- Improves physical performance, because it is important for muscle contraction;
- Prevents osteoporosis, because it helps to produce hormones that increase bone formation;
- Helps to control diabetes, because it regulates the transport of sugar;
- Decreases the risk of heart disease, as it decreases the accumulation of fatty plaques in blood vessels;
- Relieves heartburn and poor digestion, especially when used in the form of magnesium hydroxide;
- Controls blood pressure, especially in pregnant women at risk for eclampsia.

In addition, magnesium is also used in laxative medications to fight constipation and in medications that act as antacids for the stomach.

MAGNESIUM-RICH FOODS

Foods rich in magnesium are usually also high in fiber, with the main ones being whole grains, legumes, and vegetables. See the full list:
- Legumes, such as beans and lentils;
- Whole grains, such as oats, whole wheat, and brown rice;
- Fruits, such as avocado, banana, and kiwi;
- Vegetables, especially broccoli, pumpkin, and green leaves, such as kale and spinach;
- Seeds, especially the pumpkin and sunflower seeds;
- Oilseeds, such as almonds, hazelnuts, Brazil nuts, cashew nuts, peanuts;
- Milk, yogurt, and other derivatives;
- Others: coffee, meat, and chocolate.

MAGNESIUM SUPPLEMENTS

Magnesium supplements are usually recommended in cases of deficiency of this mineral, being possible to use both a multivitamin supplement in general containing magnesium and the magnesium supplement, which is normally used in the form of chelated magnesium, magnesium aspartate, magnesium citrate, magnesium lactate, or magnesium chloride.

Supplementation should be indicated by the doctor or nutritionist, as the recommended dose depends on the factor causing your deficiency, in addition, its excess can cause nausea, vomiting, hypotension, drowsiness, double vision, and weakness.

PROBIOTICS

Probiotics are foods or supplements that contain live microorganisms intended to maintain or enhance the "good" bacteria (normal microbiota) in the body. Prebiotics are foods (generally high in fiber) that act as nutrients for the human microbiota and are used with the intention of improving the balance of these microorganisms. Probiotics are found in foods like yogurt, sauerkraut, whole grains, bananas, green leafy vegetables, onions, garlic, soybeans, and artichokes. Additionally, probiotics and prebiotics are added to some foods and are available as dietary supplements.

The gut microbiota's connection to disease is being researched. The health benefits of probiotics and prebiotics currently available have not been proven conclusively.

However, side effects are uncommon, and most healthy adults can safely consume prebiotics and probiotics-containing foods. Future research could lead to more advanced probiotics with greater health benefits.

ESSENTIAL NUTRIENTS AFTER 50 YEARS

To get the most out of your 50s, you have to keep increasing your nutrient intake as you age. Once a person's body has finished going through certain changes, a series of important events occur in their bodily system, which influences many vital organs' functioning. It is critical to follow a healthy diet to help prevent the development of chronic illnesses.

Whether or not you already know this, I think you should be aware that dietary requirements change with age and lifestyle. Athletes, for example, require a higher level of carbohydrates than people who are not involved in regular physical activity. Just as is the case with nutritional needs in general, the amount of nutrients required through diet differs depending on the individual's age.

Once you have discovered the nutrients you should be concerned about, you will find out which of those nutrients are crucial in your diet because of their health effects. But if you do have any questions, please consult your trusted nutritionist.

CALCIUM

A calcium deficiency can lead to bone problems. It has been shown to help prevent bone fractures, which is why you should keep ingesting them.

However, this nutrient is much more important in women than in men. This is because, after menopause, they are more likely to develop osteoporosis due to hormonal changes.

On the other hand, it is necessary to ensure that vitamin D levels are adequate. This substance plays a key role in allowing calcium to be absorbed at the intestinal level, where it then makes its way to the bone tissue and then it must carry out its essential functions.

B12 VITAMIN

Vitamin B12 is essential in the differentiation of red blood cell lines. Anemia occurs without this compound, causing extreme fatigue and tiredness. According to a study in the Medical Clinics of North America, "megaloblastic anemia" was once known as "metaphosphate osteodystrophy".

Developing a disease like this could have a significant impact on lifestyle habits. To ensure that the requirements are met, simply include animal-based foods in the diet regularly.

PROTEIN

It has been commonly claimed that high-protein diets are bad for the liver and kidneys. However, current evidence disputes this.

Some nutrients must be increased in the diet by the age of 50 to preserve lean mass, as suggested by research. A daily protein intake of 1.4 grams per kilogram of bodyweight might be ideal.

Remember that the ingested proteins must be 50% of high biological value. All essential amino acids and a good digestibility value must be present. Also, those who are from animal-based foods exhibit both characteristics

FOODS THAT YOU SHOULD CONSIDER IN YOUR DIET AFTER 50 YEARS

It is necessary to highlight certain foods in the diet to avoid deficiencies that may negatively affect health.

MEAT AND FISH

The taste for meat and fish does diminish after age, and the preference for these meats wanes as one gets older, but it is imperative to keep up a consistent diet of meat and fish to maintain proper nutrition. These products contain high-quality proteins and essential micronutrients, like iron, that can avoid the risk of anemia.

EGGS

Eggs were once believed to increase cholesterol and raise LDL (bad cholesterol) levels, but now the myth has been debunked. Even if these foods may not influence the body's lipid profile or the risk of cardiovascular disease, they don't appear to increase cardiovascular disease risk. Also, they supply amino acids and fats which help with promoting a healthy state of well-being. Finally, they have vitamin D, a nutrient that is severely lacking in a large segment of the population. It is recommended to consume at least 5 servings of it each week.

GREEN LEAFY VEGETABLES

Green leafy vegetables are known to contain phytonutrients and vitamin C in their composition. While each element is required for proper bodily functions, it is equally important to ensure proper bodily reactions each day.

It should be noted that this vitamin is an essential nutrient that keeps the immune system in an operational state and thus keeps different infectious diseases at bay.

TIPS AND ASPECTS TO CONSIDER FOR A GOOD DIET AFTER 50 YEARS

You can still include foods as you age; however, other health strategies should be considered, such as increasing the frequency of consumption or choosing specific foods to increase intake.

PRACTICE INTERMITTENT FASTING

Fasting has been proven to improve insulin resistance and reduce fat levels in those who follow it. Most people can benefit from them, though they are not ideal for everyone. To be sure, consulting with a professional is always a good idea.

MELATONIN SUPPLEMENTS

Melatonin is a neurohormone synthesized in the pineal gland and regulating sleep-wake cycles. From the age of 50, its production drops dramatically, which can condition the quality of rest.

To avoid having the condition, you should ingest it externally. Consumption of 1.8 milligrams of the substance 30 minutes before going to sleep helps reduce the number of interruptions that happen during the night. Additionally, it is a powerful antioxidant, which has beneficial effects on the promotion of pathologies comprised of several factors.

CONSUME FERMENTED FOODS

The intestinal microbiota undergoes a variety of changes as the years go by. The change in the diversity of species that occurs over time may alter digestive function.

Thus, it is essential to consume fermented dairy, such as yogurt or kefir regularly. The good bacteria found in these foods are capable of colonizing different areas of the digestive tract. As a result, they can benefit the host's overall health.

CHAPTER 11

INTERMITTENT FASTING
AND GOOD HABITS

THE IMPORTANCE OF BREAKFAST

A good breakfast is essential for beginning the day on the right foot and having the needed energy to handle everything. How many times have we heard the importance of breakfast been preached to us? Despite that, we simply cannot eat anything. We wake up without an appetite, or in a hurry, so we do not even have the time to eat anything. This is a significant blunder.

Professionals never tire of repeating the importance of not skipping breakfast. You must remember, first of all, that you have not eaten anything in many hours, and the body needs to replenish energy. It seems contradictory, but people who eat a good breakfast have fewer weight problems; and those who do not get breakfast have problems with memory and concentration and, of course, have a bad character throughout the day.

THE IMPORTANCE OF BREAKFAST: HAVE A GOOD BREAKFAST AND START THE DAY STRONG

Breakfast represents the breaking of the fast, lays the foundations of a good diet, and benefits health. Thanks to breakfast, the body can stay strong, with higher concentration and energy levels throughout the morning.

In the case of children, the importance of breakfast is even greater, of course. Your body and brain are in full growth and are highly dependent on regular food consumption. By skipping breakfast and going for a long period without eating, the child could suffer from various physical, intellectual, and behavioral problems.

However, we often skip this meal, because we are in a hurry, out of laziness, or because of the false idea that by skipping breakfast, one can lose weight more quickly. However, a study cited in Pediatrics found that teens who ate breakfast daily had lower body mass index than teens who never ate breakfast or ate breakfast only occasionally.

WHAT CAN A BALANCED BREAKFAST INCLUDE?

Dairy products. You can choose the ones you like the most, but it is better if they are whole. Mainly milk or yogurt is ideal. They provide vitamins, proteins, and calcium.

Fruits. It is a basic element, if you also take them with skin, they give you the fiber you need. They also contain minerals, carbohydrates, and vitamins. Keep in mind that fiber has been shown to increase feelings of fullness.

Cereals or whole wheat bread. They have not only carbohydrates from which to draw energy but also fiber.

Eggs.

Meat, for example, ham. But be careful, it is not advisable to overdo this ingredient.

Coffee or herbal teas.

It is important to keep in mind that breakfast should provide about 25% of your daily caloric intake. Of course, we must try to combine the different elements in a balanced way, so that the body can absorb the necessary vitamins, fiber, carbohydrates, and minerals.

Avoid Trans Fats at Breakfast

One of the main problems in the breakfast of many people is unhealthy products, high in simple sugars and trans fats. This class of elements is capable of increasing inflammation in the body and the chances of getting sick.

Therefore, when planning a breakfast, you must include quality food, such as the ones we have mentioned. This way, you will make sure to carry out an adequate supply of nutrients to guarantee the body's proper functioning during the day.

Having a Good Breakfast Is Key

Anyway, suppose you have doubts about making a good breakfast. In that case, what products to include or how to distribute them throughout the week, it is best to consult a professional or nutritionist.

A professional in the field can help you find a good, healthy, and balanced diet. This way, you will maximize the benefits of taking care of the first meal of the day.

What Time Is It Healthiest to Eat Each Meal?

Losing or gaining weight is not just about eating healthier, but also about the times when it is done. Although it is not about following a strict schedule, except in diets prescribed by specialists, there are fundamental rules when eating certain foods.

Next, we will see some recommendations on the most appropriate times to take each food. Chrono nutrition is the science that studies the effects of nutrients depending on when they are consumed. This discipline is set to gain a lot of importance in the coming years.

It Is Healthier to Eat at Least Five Meals a Day

Today, most specialists argue that people should eat at least five times each day. That includes the traditional breakfast, lunch, and dinner, plus two snacks or snacks, between meals.

This is complemented by another idea that seems to be quite ingrained within the medical profession. They argue that the periods between one meal and another should not exceed three hours. On the contrary, overweight problems may appear or it may be difficult for us to lose the excess kilos.

The reason for this statement is that, once this time has passed, the body will notice that it is not receiving enough energy recharges and will start saving. This could cause your metabolism to slow down and not burn calories properly.

However, the most current trends are beginning to see other possibilities. One of them is intermittent fasting protocols, which are effective in improving body composition.

Breakfast

The first meal of the day has to be used to replenish all the energy used during the hours of sleep. Also, it also prepares the body for the day of physical and mental effort that is about to start.

Specialists recommend not skipping any meal and in the case of breakfast, it is essential. You have to start the day by taking the necessary nutrients.

It is understood that the healthiest breakfast consists of dairy food, fruit, and cereals. However, this is not a closed rule, it depends on each person. The important fact is that it must be as healthy as possible. As for the schedules, you should have breakfast as early as possible. It is best not to do it after 10.

Lunch at Noon

Some specialists maintain that the best time to eat the "third" (not the "second") meal of the day is between 1:00 and 3:00 p.m.

Eating high-calorie meals after 3 p.m. can be particularly counterproductive. This is because the process of digesting food becomes more inefficient so you could gain more weight. The latest research suggests that eating too early may reduce the risk of gaining fat mass.

At Night You Have to Prepare to Sleep

Just as breakfast should be forceful to gather energy for the day to begin, dinner should be the lightest of all meals of the day.

It is healthier to have an early dinner to give your body time to digest. Also, fish or lean meats are recommended, accompanied by some dairy (as long as we do not have gastric problems.)

Food intakes after 10 pm can make us gain a little more weight and, also, cause nightmares and insomnia problems.

About Desserts, Fruits, Coffee, and Snacks

Desserts are usually always in the spotlight when talking about diets, losing weight, or not gaining weight.

Some assure that they should be banished from the menu without any contemplation.

There are fewer radical opinions, which argue that they can be eaten in moderation, however, in no case, after any of the three main meals.

In the case of desserts, it is recommended to take them first thing in the morning, since before noon the body processes carbohydrates much better.

Another good time is just before starting any physical activity. Thus, you will fill the body with energy, without forcing the stomach too much.

One tip becoming fashionable is to have a piece of fruit before eating and not as a dessert. This can be a good way to decrease hunger and feeling, besides to achieving a satiating effect.

Good Hydration: as Important as Eating

There is no healthy diet if you don't consume enough water. This helps us feel more satiated, which can help us lose weight. Besides, it also contributes in a certain way to the metabolism of fats.

Specialists also recommend certain times for this:

Two glasses of water as soon as you wake up to cleanse the body.

A glass half an hour before the main meals, as well as before bathing and sleeping.

In total, you should consume between a litter and a half and two liters of water a day. However, these schedules alone do not work. We must combine them with a balanced diet and regular exercise.

Things You Can Do to Get Back to Your Ideal Weight
Avoid Consuming Sugar

It is generally known that sugary foods are a significant contributor to obesity. Conversely, since they increase the risk of diabetes, obesity, and heart disease, they also cause them.

Tips

- Replace refined sugar with healthy sweeteners like honey or stevia.
- Read the labels of the foods you buy at the grocery store and make sure they are low in sugar and saturated

fat.
- Calm your sweet tooth with "light" desserts or nuts.

EAT A GOOD BREAKFAST

Not eating a good breakfast everyday makes it difficult to regain your ideal weight. Not only have those who avoid the food run the risk of being overweight, but their physical and mental well-being also suffer.

TIPS

- Make sure you prepare a complete and balanced breakfast, which corresponds to 25% of your total daily calories.
- Eat plenty of fruits, vegetables, and complex carbohydrate sources.
- Don't forget a small helping of healthy fats and protein.

INCREASE YOUR WATER INTAKE

Water helps to improve your figure and body weight in many ways. Since much of the body is made up of this fluid, it is essential for metabolism and an optimal detoxification process.

TIPS

- Drink between 3 and 4 liters of water a day.
- If you do not want to drink only water, supplement your fluid intake with herbal teas, natural juices, or fruits rich in water.
- On hot days or when doing sports activities, increase your consumption.

GET A GOOD NIGHT'S SLEEP TO RETURN TO YOUR IDEAL WEIGHT

To successfully lose weight, ensure you do not skip any rest days. Despite appearing to be unrelated, sleep plays a central role in metabolic functions and all weight-loss-related processes.

TIPS

- Try to sleep without interruptions for 7 or 8 hours a day.
- Avoid distractions before sleeping so as not to shorten the rest period.
- Have a light dinner so that you do not have digestive discomfort when going to bed.

AVOID ZERO CARBOHYDRATE DIETS

Reducing carbohydrate consumption has interesting effects in controlling overweight. However, it is not advisable to eliminate them from the diet. These macronutrients are a major source of energy that should be incorporated into any meal plan.

TIPS

- Instead of choosing simple carbohydrates (bread, pastries, flours, etc.) opt for complex carbohydrate sources (oatmeal, brown rice, quinoa, etc.)
- Try to consume them only for breakfast and lunch.

DIVIDE THE PORTIONS OF FOOD

Large plates are not a good option for a healthy and slimming diet. While they are satisfying for the moment, they overload digestion and slow metabolism. The best option is to divide the servings by five or six meals a day.

- Eat small meals every 3-4 hours.
- Choose to have 3 main meals and 2 snacks.

REDUCE THE SALT

To return to your ideal weight, you must avoid salt. Although this condiment is commonly used in the kitchen, overconsumption affects negatively both health and figure. Too much salt causes high blood pressure, inflammation, and fluid retention.

TIPS

- Use herbs and spices to enhance the flavor.
- Do not use your favorite products if they contain a lot of sodium.

GET PHYSICAL EXERCISE

Regular physical exercise is the best complement to your diet. This type of activity starts the metabolism and optimizes the energy burn. Therefore, following a training routine or playing sports is very beneficial.

HOW TO USE INTERMITTENT FASTING BENEFITS TO BETTER YOUR LIFE

Scientists have found many advantages of intermittent fasting to reduce caloric intake for one cause or another. With this approach, the body will adjust several characteristics for the better. The real question is not if fasting can help you or not, but how it will help you and how often you should.

This fasting style has been shown to lower blood pressure and increase levels of HDL. It can help greatly with diabetes management and will also help you lose weight. All these effects sound pretty good and can be achieved with the fasting of this type. Studies carried out on several different animal species show that limiting caloric intake increases their lives by 30 percent.

Human studies show it reduces blood pressure, blood sugar, and sensitivity to insulin. With these experiments, fasting would improve a human's life if performed for an extended period. Cutting the calories by 30 percent all the time will achieve the same results, but this has been shown to cause depression and irritability. Fasting is a method offered instead of simply cutting calories and it has benefits without stress or irritability.

Intermittent fasting works out every other day by eating food. You will end up eating nearly twice as much food on the days you eat as you normally would. You still get the same number of calories but you are also getting all the benefits. It will lower the levels of stress and improve your overall health. This kind of fasting is a great way of getting into better physical condition, living a longer life, and feeling better all the time.

DIET TO REDUCE STRESS AND INCREASE HAPPINESS

Stress and our body share a strong relationship. For example, muscle tension is a reflex reaction to stress; it is the body's way of protecting itself against danger. It may feel like a little ache or something tightening in the back of your neck or lower back as you type on the computer. Headaches are a close cousin. The relationship is so strong that it has its term: stress headaches (also known as "tension pains.")

Stress even causes digestive problems as it alters the concentration of acid in the stomach that can lead to inflammation, colic, diarrhea, constipation, irritable bowel syndrome, and even peptic ulcers. Stress disrupts the body's insulin production, which can lead to diabetes and even heart attacks or strokes. Healthy diets have been shown to prevent these damaging physical effects of stress and even reverse the ageing process. Life is short, and your diet is an easy way to take control and maximize your well-being.

Eating a healthy diet will make you a more effective leader. You owe it to yourself to properly feed your body and brain, so here are four steps to creating a successful eating plan.

Give Priority to Breakfast

Starting the day well is important. You should get into the habit of eating breakfast. Skipping breakfast can make it difficult to maintain stable blood sugar levels. What you give to your body is also important. Try to choose foods high in fiber like cereals, oatmeal, whole wheat bread, and fresh fruit. High-fiber foods digest more slowly and keep you satisfied, as well as jump-start your metabolism and stabilize your blood sugar levels, allowing you to focus and reduce your anxiety and stress.

As a leader, breakfast may be the most important meal of the day, but it doesn't end there. Intermittent fasting for sugar control and weight loss can harm your mind and the relationships you have with your team. When you value the connection between your stomach and your mind, you get the most out of your day. The gift of life is quite short and fleeting.

Limit the Consumption of Refined Sugars and Processed Foods

Certain foods can harm your brain. Do not go near refined sugar. White sugar and high fructose corn syrup should be avoided. You should not give your team these foods, as you want them to be successful too.

Low-sugar diets have been shown to increase brain neurotrophic factor (BDNF), a peptide responsible for creating new neurons. This peptide makes neurons connect and combine, in addition to playing a fundamental role in neuroplasticity.

Try to avoid filling your kitchen with products high in sugar and foods with a high glycemic index such as bread, sweet drinks, and fast food. Better try fruit, honey, or maple syrup. Or better yet, go for a natural protein like soy that will help you build muscle. Refined sugars will give you a quick energy boost, but you'll soon feel like your blood sugar is on a roller coaster ride, not a fun one.

When sugar levels drop, your adrenal glands release stress hormones like cortisol. This will affect your performance as a leader. You will be more irritable in conversations; your relationships will suffer and you will not make the correct decisions that your team needs.

Include Omega-3 Fatty Acids

Omega-3 fatty acids are gifts for any leader and you deserve to include them in your diet. Nuts and seeds, including chia, flaxseed, and walnuts, are your best friends and partners. Nuts are known to protect the heart and contain antioxidants. Walnuts are particularly healthy and a rich source of omega-3 fatty acids that reduce the risk of heart attacks and bad cholesterol.

Omega-3 helps stabilize adrenal hormones and prevent them from spiking, especially when you're stressed, thus becoming a powerful antidote to stress.

Limit Your Intake of Caffeine and Alcohol

Craving caffeinated foods is natural. We all crave coffee, tea, soda, or chocolate, but it's important to recognize that these foods can affect our overall well-being. Caffeine stimulates the production of cortisol, the stress hormone. Having an occasional cup of coffee is fine, but try to avoid it before bed because it can give you insomnia. You should also think about when and how to consume alcohol. Alcohol is a depressant and sedative that alters neurotransmitters in the brain. Having a couple of beers or a couple of glasses of wine after work may sound tempting, but try not to overdo this habit because it could negatively affect your performance as a leader.

When you are stressed, it is easier to indulge in cravings and give in to impulses, facilitating drug or alcohol use as a defense mechanism. In the long term, this can result in addiction. It is best to avoid these temptations when you are experiencing high levels of stress.

Your eating habits and the level of stress you handle go hand in hand. When you're stressed, it's natural to crave comfort foods like desserts, fast food, and alcohol, but these foods can be addictive and wind you down a dead-end spiral. Fuelling your body for success will reduce stress, improve your productivity, and strengthen your relationship with your team, so keep these four steps in mind to create a high-performance eating plan.

Tips to Start a Healthy Life

- Learn something new every day. Healthy entrepreneurs are eternal dreamers: They work hard, play hard and think hard. They love to read, listen to audiobooks, and absorb as much knowledge as possible. They educate themselves on topics relevant to their business and also seek knowledge of other types. They know that healthy behaviors have a direct impact on their business.

- Set goals and create systems to achieve them: Healthy entrepreneurs also understand that knowledge without application is the fastest path to failure. They go beyond learning-they apply. They realize that daily journeys and steps are the only way to achieve goals.

- If you want to make the most of your free time, spend it wisely: It is estimated the average person spends three hours per day watching television. That is a very kind thing of you to do, but please do not be that kind of person. To stay healthy, you should concentrate on growing your business, taking care of yourself and your family, and making the world a better place. Another piece of advice is to spend time or engage in meditation to gain a better sense of your goals.

- Make exercise a priority. A healthy body helps cultivate a healthy mind: An adult should exercise 2.5 hours a week or more with moderate to intense aerobic activity and two intensive training sessions a week. Even if you are very busy, find 10 minutes here and there. Doing so will help you relieve stress and get endorphins to overcome your business challenges.

- Eat less junk food. Think of food as fuel: The higher the quality of fuel you put in your tank, the better you will perform. You don't need to go on a diet to eat healthily. Only eat more real foods (that come from nature), instead of processed and fast food. Doing so will improve your energy level and mood, among other benefits.

- Get more sleep. All entrepreneurs experience sleepless nights, morning meetings, and last-minute deliveries. But a healthy entrepreneur knows that sleep is essential to their success. Whether you're getting up early and getting big projects done in the morning or you're hopelessly awake, find a consistent sleep routine and stick with it. Don't underestimate the power of a good nap to recharge your brain, either.

- Create a balance in your life: Healthy entrepreneurs treat their health as a lifestyle. You can't put a Band-Aid on a bad Business Plan, just like you can't eat healthy for a week and hope to lose weight. Successful entrepreneurs adopt a healthy lifestyle: They work smart, they don't work anymore.

CHAPTER 12

Let's talk about the most typical myths about intermittent fasting, especially concerning fitness.

If you want to gain muscle mass in the world of fitness, you have to make many meals to accelerate the metabolism, incorporate protein in each of them, and do not forget to drink your post-workout shake.

Of course, many fitness gurus will never recommend you perform fasting workouts for the possible loss of muscle mass, so let's shed some light on it.

Fasting Periods Reduce Metabolism

In general, there is an excessive and irrational fear that our metabolism will slow down. In this book we have already seen the real impact of caloric restriction and weight loss on metabolism.

Performing fasting periods does not reduce our basal metabolism, yes, it has been repeated throughout life that if you skip breakfast your metabolism is reduced, your body goes into saving mode and you will accumulate body fat.

But this statement is false, skipping breakfast does not reduce metabolism.

On the other hand, in several studies, it has been observed that fasting does not reduce metabolism either. In fact, in this study it was observed that fasting increased the levels of norepinephrine, a catecholamine with different physiological functions, increasing metabolism.

Another reason for criticizing intermittent fasting is the frequency of meals.

Some people say that intermittent fasting is not a good option to lose body fat because the number of made meals is reduced, which can hurt metabolism.

We know that there is no difference between making 3 or 6 meals when losing body fat. This study also reaches the same conclusion, making more meals a day does not translate into a greater loss of body fat.

On the other hand, some studies conclude that alternating fasting days is more effective for losing weight than traditional caloric restriction. In contrast, in others, it has been observed that it is not superior after one year of follow-up.

The nutritional strategy to follow depends on the person. As always, you have to individualize; some people will adapt better to fasting and the results will be better.

But it must be made clear that fasting does not reduce metabolism. In any case, the short-term impact would be positive.

Fasting Causes Loss of Muscle Mass

Fasting not only reduces your basal metabolism but also makes you lose muscle mass as many keep repeating today.

Although caloric restriction (especially if the caloric deficit is very aggressive) can lead to a loss of muscle mass, this loss of muscle mass will be greatly reduced if we include strength training and enough protein in the diet. If we add fast to this equation, the result remains the same. If you perform heavy strength workouts, include enough protein in your diet, and control the calories you are consuming, the loss of muscle mass will be minimal.

In different studies, it has been observed that it is possible to lose body fat and maintain muscle mass while following a fasting protocol.

It has been observed that in people who practice Ramadan (with experience in training) there is a loss of body weight, but not muscle tissue.

Fasting Increases the Feeling of Hunger So That You Will Eat More

In many studies, there has been an increase in the feeling of hunger.

That is, in general, fasting does seem to increase the sensation of hunger. Still, it has not been observed that this contributes to an increase in caloric intake throughout the day. The opposite has been observed, performing 1 day of fasting translates into a 30% reduction in caloric intake the next 3 days, 30%.

Besides, under my personal experience, there is a period of adaptation; the feeling of hunger is reduced as you practice more intermittent fasting. My recommendation is that while you do it, try to be active. Some exercise is fine. Although if you are starting, it is better to start progressively.

Fasting Improves Athletic Performance

Another of the supposed benefits is that performing fasting workouts improves athletic performance.

The reality is that there is no scientific evidence to affirm that fasting improves athletic performance. The studies available today contradict this claim. Training on an empty stomach is not a useful strategy to improve performance.

In fact, and it is important to mention that, in some studies, the maximum that was achieved was to maintain the performance, and not always. In several of the sports, performance was reduced (although it could be due to other factors).

What Happens When You Don't Eat For 24 Hours? Myth vs. Reality

Myth 1: Your Metabolism Slows Down

This idea has its origin in studies with mice, but there are two problems:

A mouse has a short life (2-3 years). A fast of a day in a mouse would perhaps equal more than a week in a human.

Mice have very little fat and are more sensitive to caloric deficits. On the contrary, humans are mammals with more% fat.

Interestingly, in us, fasting causes a slight increase in metabolism, partly because of the release of norepinephrine and orexin. It is an evolutionary adaptation: motivation to go hunting.

Of course, a prolonged fast will slow the metabolism. It is logical, knowing that leptin takes several days to reduce enough the hypothalamus tendency to react, regulating downward energy expenditure.

As we saw in this book, what slows down the metabolism is precisely a prolonged period of a hypocaloric diet, just what they recommend.

Myth 2: Burn Muscle

When your body has consumed all the amino acids in the blood and stored glycogen, it start using protein stores, your muscles, to convert them into glucose (via gluconeogenesis). You should avoid this process, but fortunately, it does not happen in the first 24 hours of fasting. A couple of examples:

A study concluded that intermittent fasting retains more muscle mass than a traditional hypocaloric approach (with similar fat loss).

Another study with intermittent fasting in obese adults found that it is effective for weight loss, even increasing muscle mass. This study also compared intermittent fasting with a high-fat approach (45% of total calories) against another moderate in fat (25% of total calories). The high fat achieved greater muscle gain and fat loss. Interesting.

One possible limitation of these studies is that they are performed in overweight people, and we know that fat protects the muscle.

What would happen in people with a lot of muscle and low fat?

According to this study in Muslim bodybuilders, fasting during the month of Ramadan does not result in loss of muscle mass. Women who trained strength with intermittent fasting (16/8) gained the same amount of muscle as those who did more meals, but they lost some more fat.

It may be due in part to the increase in growth hormone generated by fasting, the protective role of autophagy, and the reduction of myostatin, which inhibits muscle development.

Supplement companies invest a lot of money in promoting the need to ingest 20g of protein every 3 hours. Their dream would be for everyone to drink protein shakes on snacks. It is not necessary.

But more is not better; a prolonged fast is dangerous for the muscle. Your tolerance level will depend on the accumulated glycogen and physical activity performed, but in general, I do not recommend frequent fasting for more than 24-36 hours. Run away from detox diets for a week, for example.

MYTH 3: LOW SUGAR

The body is designed to maintain the proper level of blood glucose. When you eat you produce insulin to store excess glucose. When you fast you produce glucagon to release stored glucose. Eating frequently to control blood glucose externally is not necessary. You can dedicate your time to more productive things.

Intermittent fasting helps restore sensitivity to a greater extent than classical calorie restriction in people with insulin resistance.

In another study, people with type II diabetes responded better to two large meals a day than six small ones. We also know that intermittent fasting is effective against metabolic problems.

MYTH 4: YOU WILL NOT GIVE UP IN TRAINING

The impact of fasting on performance depends on many factors, such as the type of physical activity, the duration of fasting, and the level of adaptation. Still, there are many examples where this loss of performance does not materialize, once adopted.

Reviews of studies in Muslim athletes during Ramadan show inconsistent results. Resistance tests are most affected, but it is necessary to consider that during Ramadan the fluids are also restricted during the day, so it is difficult to know what effect is due to fasting and which is due to daily dehydration. In any case, the variations are small.

The truth is that fasting training (with low glycogen) favors adaptations that would not occur if you always train with full reserves.

And finally, a recent study in strength athletes demonstrates that an intermittent fasting strategy not only maintains muscle performance and gains, but is more effective in losing fat. The same happens in women this study concludes.

MYTH 5: YOU WILL BE HUNGRY, HEADACHES, AND IRRITATION

It is possible that all this happens the first time. Like everything, it is a matter of adaptation.

But there is much evidence against distributing food in many small intakes:

A study concluded that increasing the frequency of meals increases hunger; while another suggested that it can promote a higher caloric intake.

My experience: the most important thing to improve adherence (and therefore success) is to be satiated when you eat. If you eat 1,800 calories a day and divide it into 6 intakes, you have 300 calories left over. Result: constant hunger. Compressing the feeding window reduces appetite.

Regarding irritation, it is subjective, but some studies indicate that intermittent fasting improves mood and symptoms of depression and improves mental alertness.

Personally, it would irritate me much more to have to prepare six meals a day and never be satiated. Intermittent fasting represents great mental and time release.

MYTH 6: YOU WILL GAIN WEIGHT

Simply absurd. Multiple studies show that intermittent fasting helps you lose fat better than classic hypocaloric diets. Recent reviews already recognize it as an effective strategy to lose weight.

The justification of some is that by skipping one meal you will accumulate hunger and you will eat twice as much at the next meal, but we know that does not happen.

CHAPTER 13

RECIPES BREAKFASTS

1. Perfect Hard-Boiled Eggs In The Easiest Manner

Prep Time: 2 minutes
Cook Time: 20 minutes
Servings: 2 people

Ingredients:
- 6 eggs
- Water

Directions:
- In a medium saucepan, crack the eggs.
- 1" above the eggs, cover with water.
- Place on high heat on the stovetop.
- Bring the water to a boil. Remove from heat and cover immediately.
- Allow for 18-20 minutes of resting time.
- Holding the pot on a slant, pour cold tap water into the saucepan, allowing the hot water to escape.
- Allow eggs to rest in cold water for 1-2 minutes before peeling.

Nutrient value: Per serving
- Calories: 71 kcal
- Carbohydrates: 0 g
- Protein: 6 g
- Fat: 4 g

2. Mix Trail

Prep Time: 2 minutes

Cook Time: 0 minutes
Servings: 6 people

Ingredients:
- almonds, 230 g (raw)
- Sunflower seeds, 230 g (raw)
- Raisins, 230 g
- dried apricot, 120 g (unsulphured, chopped)
- flaked coconut 60 g (optional)
- 60 g chocolate or 60 g carob chips

- **Directions:**
- Combine all ingredients in a big container, cover, and shake!
- Keep the container airtight.
- Refrigerate or freeze to preserve the vital fatty acid characteristics.

Nutrient value: Whole recipe
- Calories: 371 kcal
- Carbohydrates: 35 g
- Protein: 10 g
- Fat: 24 g

3. Bowl Of Savory Oats

Prep Time: 10 minutes
Cook Time: 30 minutes
Servings: 4 people

Ingredients:
- 225 g halved Brussels sprouts

- 450 g container cubed butternut squash
- 15 ml extra virgin olive oil
- 3 g salt (distributed)
- 3 g black pepper (distributed)
- 15 g unsalted butter
- 120 g finely chopped onion
- Quaker Old Fashioned Oats, 450 g
- 450 ml liquid
- 120 g Sharp Cheddar cheese, shredded
- 4 quail eggs
- 2 cooked turkey bacon strips, crumbled

Directions:
- Preheat oven to 204□ C.
- Using parchment paper, line a large baking sheet.
- Toss the butternut squash, Brussels sprouts, chopped onion, olive oil, salt, and black pepper in a large mixing bowl and transfer to a baking sheet.
- Bake the vegetables for 20 to 22 minutes, or until tender and golden brown.
- Melt the butter in a medium pot over medium heat while the vegetables roast. Cook for 30 seconds to toast the oats.
- Bring the water to a boil, then reduce to a low heat.
- Reduce the heat to low and continue to cook for 8 to 10 minutes, or until the oats reach a thick consistency, adding more water as needed.
- Season with the remaining salt and black pepper, then fold in the shredded cheese.
- Maintain your body temperature.
- Cook eggs sunny-side up or over easy in a large greased nonstick skillet.
- Scoop oats into a bowl, top with veggies, an egg, and bacon crumbles, and serve.

Nutrient value: Whole recipe
- Calories: 460 kcal
- Carbohydrates: 56 g
- Protein: 19g
- Fat: 17 g

4. THE BUDDHA BOWL

Prep Time: 10 minutes
Cook Time: 15 minutes
Servings: 2 people

Ingredients:
- 2 poached pastured eggs
- 2 precooked Paleo sausages (we used a spicy lamb sausage)
- 250 g riced cauliflower
- Cooking with grass-fed ghee
- 1 avocado, sliced
- 1/4 cucumber, sliced
- 2 handfuls lightly steamed organic leafy greens
- Garnish with fresh herbs, sliced chilli, sliced spring onions, a wedge of lemon, and salt and pepper to taste.

Directions:
- Melt butter in a frying pan over medium heat.
- Allow 20 g of ghee to melt throughout the pan. Cook until the cauliflower rice is done to your liking.
- Arrange the leafy greens on a plate or in a large bowl.
- When the cauliflower rice is done, serve it with the leafy greens.
- Reheat the sausages in the same frying pan.
- Meanwhile, arrange the avocado, sliced cucumber, and poached eggs on top of the cauliflower rice and leafy greens.
- When the sausages are done, add them to the bowl with the rest of the ingredients.
- Garnish with your choice of garnishes, then serve and enjoy!

Nutrient value: Per serving
- Calories: 323 kcal
- Carbohydrates: 13 g
- Protein: 25 g
- Fat: 40 g

Prep Time: 5 minutes
Cook Time: 10 minutes
Servings: 3 people

Ingredients:
- 50g (half a cup) coconut flour
- 3 g baking soda
- 10 ml melted coconut oil
- 4 organic, pasture-raised eggs, room temp.
- 3 ml vanilla extract
- 3 g cinnamon, Ceylon
- 250 g of coconut cream (the thick part of canned coconut cream, unsweetened)
- 120 ml unsweetened almond milk
- Himalayan salt, 2 g
- Grass-fed Cooking using ghee or coconut oil

Directions:
- In a high-powered blender, combine all ingredients except the ghee and process until well combined, scraping down the sides as needed.
- Heat ghee in a medium skillet over medium heat until it coats the pan.
- When the pan is hot, add half batter into it.
- Cook the batter until golden on one side, then turn and cook until golden on the other (note: Thicker pancakes will take longer to cook). Set aside and continue to cook until no batter is left.
- Serve heated coconut flour pancakes with grass-fed ghee, fruit, or other keto-friendly toppings.

Nutrient value: Per serving
- Calories: 244 kcal
- Carbohydrates: 5 g
- Protein: 5 g
- Fat: 23 g

Prep Time: 10 minutes
Cook Time: 15 minutes
Servings: 2 people

Ingredients:
- 450 g cauliflower, grated
- 30 g coconut flour
- 4 eggs,
- 3 g salt
- 15 g powdered psyllium husk (Use a mold-free brand, such as this one.)
- Smoked salmon, avocado, herbs, spinach, and olive oil (see post for more suggestions)

Directions:
- Preheat the oven to 176°C.
- Use parchment paper to line a pizza tray or a sheet pan.
- Mix all ingredients except the toppings in a mixing bowl until well blended. Allow coconut flour and psyllium husk to absorb liquid and thicken for 5 minutes.
- Pour the morning pizza base onto the pan with care. Form it into a circular, even pizza crust using your hands.
- Bake for 15 minutes, or until golden brown and cooked through.
- Remove the morning pizza from the oven and top with your preferred toppings. Serve hot.

Nutrient value: Per serving
- Calories: 454 kcal
- Carbohydrates: 26 g
- Protein: 22 g
- Fat: 31 g

Prep Time: 10 minutes
Cook Time: 25 minutes
Servings: 4 people

Ingredients:
- two eggs
- 120 g almond flour
- 120 g coconut shredded

- 120 g almonds, sliced
- 120 g toasted pecans
- 120 g pumpkin seeds
- 12 0 g chocolate chips (sugar-free)
- 75 g toasted almond butter
- 75 g of granulated monk fruit-erythritol blend
- 30 g ground flax meal
- 7 g Bulletproof Collagen Protein in Vanilla
- 20 g cinnamon
- 20 g ginger powder
- 15 ml vanilla extract

Directions:
- Preheat the oven to 176°C.
- Line two baking sheets with parchment paper.
- In a mixing dish, combine all cookie ingredients.
- Coat your hands in coconut oil and roll the mixture into balls. Place them on the baking sheets that have been lined with parchment paper and press them into flat, even cookies.
- Place the baking tray in the oven and bake for 20-25 minutes, or until golden and cooked through.
- Remove the cookies from the oven and set aside to cool.
- For a keto-friendly breakfast, serve with a hot cup of Bulletproof Coffee!

Nutrient value: Per serving
- Calories: 289 kcal
- Carbohydrates: 17 g
- Protein: 8 g
- Fat: 29 g

---

8. Smoked Salmon Breakfast Sandwich

Prep Time: 5 minutes
Cook Time: 10 minutes
 Servings: 4 people

Ingredients:
- 60 ml coconut oil
- 8 slices of your choice of sandwich vessel (like Cauliflower Sandwich Thins)
- smoked salmon, 110 g
- 225 g fresh spinach
- 2 whole pasture-raised eggs or 60 g organic powdered eggs
- 60 ml water
- 2 garlic cloves or 7 g garlic powder
- half a lemon

Directions:
- If you're using powdered eggs, hydrate them in water first.
- Allow for a 5-minute resting period after stirring.
- Meanwhile, heat the burner to medium.
- 30 ml coconut oil in a pan
- Toast both sides of the sandwich bread.
- Mince the garlic cloves while the bread is browning.
- Once all of the slices have been roasted, add the remaining 2 tablespoons coconut oil to the pan.
- Cook the garlic for 1-2 minutes.
- Cook for 2-3 minutes, or until the spinach is wilted.
- Add the eggs. Cook for 2-3 minutes, stirring gently, until set.
- Finish with a squirt of lemon juice.
- Toast with smoked salmon and garlic spinach scramble.
- Eat!

Nutrient value: Per serving
- Calories: 130 kcal
- Carbohydrates: 0g
- Protein: 3 g
- Fat: 5 g

---

9. Breakfast With Scrambled Eggs

Prep Time: 2 minutes
Cook Time: 5 minutes
 Servings: 1 people

Ingredients:

- 1 large egg
- 60 g of egg whites
- 500 g cheddar cheese
- Avocado (15 g)
- 120 g thinly sliced mushrooms

Directions:

- Whisk together the egg and the egg whites.
- Spray a skillet with cooking spray and cook until the mixture is no longer runny.
- Sauté the mushrooms in a separate skillet with butter-flavored cooking spray.
- Shred cheese and slice avocado.
- Melt the cheese on top of the eggs.
- Cooked mushrooms and sliced avocado should be added.

Nutrient value: Per serving

- Calories: 263 kcal
- Carbohydrates: 1 g
- Protein: 5 g
- Fat: 5g

10. English Breakfast With Low Carbs

Prep Time: 5minutes
Cook Time: 5 minutes
Servings: 1 people

Ingredients:

- 1 eggs,
- 20 g bacon,
- 2 sausages,
- 30 g mushrooms
- 1 sliced avocado,
- 1 roasted tomatoes and
- 30 g wilted spinach

Directions:

- Make your usual breakfast of eggs, bacon, sausage, mushrooms, and black pudding.
- Remove the bread, hash browns, and any other high-carbohydrate products.
- If desired, top with sliced avocado, roasted tomatoes, and wilted spinach.

Nutrient value: Per serving

- Calories: 69 kcal
- Carbohydrates: 0 g
- Protein: 2 g
- Fat: 5 g

11. The French Omelet

Prep Time: 10minutes
Cook Time: 10 minutes
Servings: 3 people

Ingredients:

- three eggs
- 4 big egg whites
- 75 ml fat-free milk
- 2 g pepper
- 2 g salt
- 75 g well cooked cubed ham
- 15 g finely sliced onion
- 3 g chopped green pepper
- 75 g reduced-fat cheddar cheese, shredded

Directions:

- Combine the first five ingredients in a mixing bowl.
- Over medium heat, heat a 10-inch skillet sprayed with cooking spray.
- Mix in the egg mixture.
- The mixture should instantly set at the edges.
- Push cooked sections toward the centre as the eggs set, allowing uncooked eggs to flow underneath.
- When the eggs have thickened and there is no longer any liquid egg, top one half with the other ingredients.
- Cut the omelette in half.
- To serve, cut in half.

Nutrient value: Per serving

- Calories: 186 kcal

- Carbohydrates: 1 g
- Protein: 22 g
- Fat: 9 g

---

12. FRITTATA WITH FETA

Prep Time: 10 minutes
Cook Time: 15 minutes
Servings: 3 people

Ingredients:
- 1 finely sliced green onion
- 1 minced tiny garlic clove
- two huge eggs
- 120 g egg replacer
- 60 g crumbled feta cheese (divided)
- 100 g chopped plum tomato
- 4 thin avocado slices, peeled
- 30 g sour cream (reduced fat)

Directions:
- Heat a 6-inch nonstick skillet over medium heat, lightly greased.
- Cook until the onion and garlic are soft.
- Combine the eggs, egg substitute, and 45 g feta cheese in a mixing bowl.
- Pour the egg mixture into the skillet (mixture should set immediately at edges).
- Cook, covered, for 4-6 minutes, or until nearly set.
- Finish with the remaining feta cheese and tomato.
- Cook, covered, for 2-3 minutes longer, or until the eggs are completely set.
- Allow for a 5-minute resting period.
- Serve with avocado and sour cream, cut in half.

Nutrient value: Per serving
- Calories: 203 kcal
- Carbohydrates: 5 g
- Protein: 17 g
- Fat: 12 g

---

13. FRITTATA WITH BACON AND ASPARAGUS

Prep Time: 10 minutes
Cook Time: 25 minutes
Servings: 6 people

Ingredients:
- Bacon, 350 g.
- 450 g fresh asparagus, sliced (cut into 1/2-inch pieces)
- 250 g finely chopped onion
- 2 minced garlic cloves
- 10 big eggs, beaten
- 60 g parsley, minced
- 2 g of seasoned salt
- 1 g pepper
- 1 large, thinly sliced tomato
- 250 g cheddar cheese, shredded

Directions:
- Cook bacon until crisp in a 9- or 10-inch oven-proof skillet.
- Drain, saving some amount of the drippings.
- Heat the conserved drippings over medium-high heat.
- Sauté the asparagus, onion, and garlic until the onion is soft.
- Set aside a third of the bacon crumbles.
- Combine the leftover bacon, eggs, parsley, salt, and pepper in a large mixing bowl.
- Pour the egg mixture into the skillet and swirl to combine.
- Top with the reserved bacon, tomato, and cheese.
- Cook, covered, over medium-low heat for 10-15 minutes, or until the eggs are nearly set. Preheat the broiler and position the skillet 6 inches from the fire.
- Broil for 2 minutes, or until lightly browned.
- Serve right away.

Nutrient value: Per Piece
- Calories: 344 kcal
- Carbohydrates: 5 g
- Protein: 24 g
- Fat: 23 g

Prep Time: 5 minutes
Cook Time: 15 minutes
Servings: 4 people

Ingredients:
*   120 g finely chopped onion
*   1 minced jalapeno pepper
*   15 ml of canola oil
*   6 big, lightly beaten eggs
*   6 cooked and crumbled bacon strips
*   1 sliced small tomato
*   1 avocado, sliced into 1-inch slices
*   250 g Monterey Jack cheese, shredded
*   Season with salt and pepper to taste.
*   Optional salsa

Directions:
*   Cook onion and jalapeno in oil in a large skillet until tender; remove with a slotted spoon and set aside.
*   Pour the eggs into the same skillet; cover and simmer for 3-4 minutes over low heat.
*   Sprinkle with the onion mixture, bacon, tomato, avocado, and half a cup of the cheese.
*   Season with salt and pepper to taste.
*   Fold the omelette in half and place it on top of the filling.
*   Cook for 3-4 minutes, or until the eggs are set.
*   Finish with the remaining cheese.
*   If preferred, serve with salsa.

Nutrient value: Per piece
*   Calories: 390 kcal
*   Carbohydrates: 6 g
*   Protein: 23 g
*   Fat: 21 g

Prep Time: 25 minutes
Cook Time: 20 minutes

Servings: 6 people
Ingredients:
*   8 medium eggs
*   a third of a cup heavy whipping cream
*   120 g grated Romano cheese,
*   2 g teaspoon salt,
*   75 ml olive oil, split
*   340 g fresh mushrooms, sliced
*   1 medium onion, cut in half and thinly sliced
*   30 g fresh basil, minced
*   2 minced garlic cloves
*   1 g black pepper
*   220 g Mascarpone ricotta

Directions:
*   Whisk together the eggs, cream, 60 g Romano cheese, and 3 g salt in a large mixing dish.
*   30 ml oil, heated in a 10-inch skillet over medium-high heat
*   Cook and stir in the mushrooms and onion until soft.
*   Cook and stir for 1 minute more after adding the basil, garlic, pepper, and remaining salt. Transfer to a mixing bowl and toss in the mascarpone and remaining Romano cheese.
*   1 5 ml oil, heated over medium-high heat in the same pan
*   150 ml of the egg mixture should be added.
*   The mixture should instantly set at the edges.
*   Push cooked sections toward the centre as the eggs set, allowing uncooked eggs to flow underneath.
*   Allow to stand for 5-7 minutes, covered, or until completely set.
*   Transfer to a serving tray, cover with foil, and keep warm.
*   Repeat with the remaining egg mixture to make two more frittatas, using the remaining oil as needed.
*   Layer half of the mushroom mixture on top of one frittata on a serving plate.
*   Layers should be repeated.
*   Finish with the leftover frittata.
*   Cut the potatoes into wedges.

Nutrient value: Per piece

- Calories: 468 kcal
- Carbohydrates: 5 g
- Protein: 20 g
- Fat: 44 g

---

16. Frittata With Zucchini And Gouda In A Skillet

Prep Time: 10 minutes
Cook Time: 20 minutes
Servings: 6 people

Ingredients:
- six huge eggs
- 30 ml 2% milk
- 15 g fresh oregano, diced
- 2 g of salt
- 1 g.black pepper
- 10 g melted butter
- 2 medium zucchini, thinly sliced, 220 g each
- 1 medium sliced onion
- 30 ml olive oil
- 1 medium diced tomato
- 250 g Gouda cheese, shredded
- 30 g fresh basil, minced

Directions:
- Set aside the first five ingredients. Melt butter in a large nonstick skillet over medium heat.
- Mix in the zucchini and onion.
- Cook for 6-8 minutes, or until the vegetables are soft; remove from the heat.
- Heat the oil in the same skillet over medium heat.
- Mix in the egg mixture.
- Cook until the egg is set, gently raising the edges of the cooked egg to allow the liquid to run below.
- Serve with the zucchini mixture, diced tomato, and cheese on top.
- Cook, covered, for 2-3 minutes, or until the cheese is melted.
- Garnish with basil.

Nutrient value: Per piece
- Calories: 238 kcal
- Carbohydrates: 5 g
- Protein: 15 g
- Fat: 19 g

17. Florentine Egg Casserole

Prep Time: 20 minutes
Cook Time: 30 minutes
Servings: 12 people

Ingredients:
- 450 g pork sausage in bulk
- 30 g melted butter
- 1 big sliced onion
- 250 g fresh sliced mushrooms
- 1 frozen chopped spinach box (250 g), thawed and pressed dry
- 12 extra-large eggs
- 2 L Milk with 2% fat
- 250 g Swiss cheese, shredded
- 250 g sharp cheddar cheese, shredded
- 2 g paprika

Directions:
- Preheat the oven to 176□ C.
- Cook sausage in a large skillet over medium heat until no longer pink, 6-8 minutes, breaking it up into crumbles; drain and transfer to a greased 13x9-inch baking dish.
- Melt butter in the same skillet over medium-high heat.
- Cook and stir for 3-5 minutes, or until the onion and mushrooms are soft.
- Mix in the spinach.
- Serve the veggie mixture on top of the sausage.
- Whisk eggs and milk together in a large mixing basin until smooth; pour egg mixture over vegetables.
- Garnish with the cheeses and paprika.
- Bake for 30-35 minutes, uncovered, or until the centre is set and a thermometer inserted into the centre reads 73°C.

- Allow to stand for 10 minutes before serving.

Nutrient value: Per piece
- Calories: 271 kcal
- Carbohydrates: 6 g
- Protein: 20 g
- Fat: 16g

-----

18. SCRAMBLED SPINACH-MUSHROOM EGGS

Prep Time: 5 minutes
Cook Time: 10 minutes
Servings: 2 people

Ingredients:
- two huge eggs
- 2 egg whites, big
- 1 g pepper
- 1 g salt
- 15 g butter
- 120 g fresh mushrooms, thinly sliced
- 120 g chopped fresh baby spinach
- 30 g provolone cheese, shredded

Directions:
- In a small mixing dish, combine the eggs, egg whites, salt, and pepper.
- Melt butter in a small nonstick skillet over medium-high heat.
- Cook and stir for 3-4 minutes, or until the mushrooms are soft.
- Cook and stir in the spinach until it is wilted.
- Turn the heat down to medium.
- Cook and whisk the egg mixture until the eggs have thickened and no liquid egg remains.
- Mix in the cheese.

Nutrient value: Per serving
- Calories: 162 kcal
- Carbohydrates: 2 g
- Protein: 15 g
- Fat: 11 g

19. QUICHE CUPS WITH BROCCOLI

Prep Time: 10 minutes
Cook Time: 15 minutes
Servings: 6 people

Ingredients:
- 250 g fresh broccoli, chopped
- 250 g pepper jack cheese, shredded
- 6 big, lightly beaten eggs
- 100 g heavy whipping cream
- 120 g bacon drippings
- 1 minced shallot
- 1 g salt
- 1 g pepper

Directions:
- Preheat the oven to 176 C.
- Divide the broccoli and cheese among 12 muffin cups that have been oiled.
- Pour the remaining ingredients into the cups after whisking them together.
- Bake for 15-20 minutes, or until the cheese is melted.

Nutrient value: Per serving (2 cups)
- Calories: 291 kcal
- Carbohydrates: 4 g
- Protein: 16 g
- Fat: 24 g

-----

20. BREAKFAST CASSEROLE WITH GREEK FLAVORS

Prep Time: 35 minutes
Cook Time: 45 minutes
Servings: 6 people

Ingredients:
- 220 g casing-free Italian turkey sausage links
- 120 g green pepper, chopped
- 1 chopped shallot
- 250 g rinsed, drained, and diced water-packed ar-

tichoke hearts
- 250 g fresh broccoli, chopped
- 100 g chopped sun-dried tomatoes (not packaged in oil)
- six huge eggs
- 6 egg whites, big
- 45 ml fat-free milk
- 7 g Italian seasoning
- 1 g garlic powder
- 1 g pepper
- 75 g feta cheese, crumbled

Directions:
- Preheat the oven to 176☐ C.
- Cook sausage, green pepper, and shallot in a large skillet over medium heat until sausage is no longer pink, 8-10 minutes, breaking up sausage into chunks; drain.
- Pour the mixture into an 8-inch square baking dish sprayed with cooking spray. Serve with artichokes, broccoli, and sun-dried tomatoes on top.
- In a large mixing bowl, combine eggs, egg whites, milk, and seasonings; pour over top.
- Garnish with feta.
- 45-50 minutes, uncovered, until a knife inserted into the centre comes out clean.
- Allow to stand for 10 minutes before serving.

Nutrient value: Per piece
- Calories: 179 kcal
- Carbohydrates: 7 g
- Protein: 17 g
- Fat: 9 g

CHAPTER 14

RECIPES APPETIZERS AND SNACKS

1. Kabobs With Chilled Chicken And Cheese

Prep Time: 20 minutes
Cook Time: 5 minutes
Servings: 8 people

Ingredients:
*   2 g of salt
*   2 g chilli powder
*   220 g boneless skinless chicken breast, diced
*   1 g pepper
*   15 ml balsamic vinegar
*   30 ml olive oil
*   140 g cubes part-skim melted mozzarella cheese
*   16 cherry tomatoes or grape tomatoes

Directions:
*   Rub chicken cubes with salt, chilli powder, and pepper.
*   Transfer to a large mixing bowl.
*   Toss in the vinegar to coat.
*   Refrigerate for 3-4 hours, covered.
*   Drain the chicken, reserving the marinade.
*   Heat the oil in a large skillet over medium heat.
*   Cook until the chicken is no longer pink.
*   Allow to cool slightly. Thread chicken, cheese, and tomatoes onto wooden skewers in alternate directions.
*   Serve chilled.

Nutrient value: Per piece

*   Calories: 93 kcal
*   Carbohydrates: 4 g
*   Protein: 13 g
*   Fat: 4 g

---

2. Deviled Eggs With Bacon And Cheddar

Prep Time: 10 minutes
Cook Time: 20 minutes
Servings: 10 people

Ingredients:
*   12 big hard-boiled eggs
*   110 g mayonnaise
*   4 cooked and crumbled bacon strips
*   30 g finely grated cheddar cheese
*   15 ml mustard honey
*   1 g pepper

Directions:
*   Cut the eggs in half lengthwise, remove the yolks, and set the whites aside.
*   Mash the yolks in a small bowl.
*   Combine the mayonnaise, bacon, cheese, mustard, and pepper in a mixing bowl.
*   Fill egg whites with stuffing or pipe with a pastry bag.
*   Refrigerate until ready to serve.

Nutrient value: Per piece
- Calories: 79 kcal
- Carbohydrates: 1 g
- Protein: 10 g
- Fat: 4 g

---

3. Lime With Spiced Hot Chipotle Spinach And Artichoke Dip

Prep Time: 10 minutes
Cook Time: 20 minutes
Servings: 4 people

Ingredients:
- 450 g mozzarella cheese, shredded
- 220 g softened cream cheese
- 120 g mayonnaise
- 120 g Parmesan cheese, grated
- 2 finely chopped chipotle chiles in adobo sauce
- 60 ml lime juice
- 15 ml grated lime zest
- 1 g kosher salt
- 1 g pepper
- 400 g drained and finely chopped water-packed artichoke hearts
- 1 frozen chopped spinach box (350 g), thawed and pressed dry
- 1 large garlic clove, neatly chopped 3 green onions, chopped
- Baked pita chips, tortilla chips, sliced French bread baguette, or different crackers are optional.

Directions:
- Preheat the oven to 204°C.
- Combine the mozzarella cheese, cream cheese, mayonnaise, and 60 g grated Parmesan cheese in a mixing bowl.
- Mix in the following 9 components.
- Pour into a deep-dish pie pan and top with the remaining Parmesan.
- Bake for 20-25 minutes, or until golden brown and bubbling.

- Serve with pita or tortilla chips, baguette pieces, or crackers as desired.

Nutrient value: Per serving
- Calories: 164 kcal
- Carbohydrates: 3 g
- Protein: 7 g
- Fat: 14 g

---

4. Miniature Frittatas De Spinach

Prep Time: 10 minutes
Cook Time: 20 minutes
Servings: 8 people

Ingredients:
- 250 g ricotta cheese (whole milk)
- 100 g Parmesan cheese, grated
- 75 g fresh mushrooms, chopped
- 1 frozen chopped spinach box (220 g), thawed and pressed dry
- a single huge egg
- 2 g dried oregano
- 1 g salt
- 1 g pepper
- 24 pepperoni slices

Directions:
- Preheat the oven to 195°C.
- Combine the first 8 ingredients in a small bowl.
- Fill each of the 24 greased mini-muffin cups three-quarters full with the cheese mixture.
- Bake for 20-25 minutes, or until the centre is completely set.
- To loosen frittatas, carefully run a knife over the sides of muffin cups.
- Serve hot.

Nutrient value: Per piece
- Calories: 128 kcal
- Carbohydrates: 4 g
- Protein: 10 g
- Fat: 9 g

Prep Time: 5 minutes
Cook Time: 15 minutes
Servings: 8 people

Ingredients:
• Boats with Avocado and Crab 5 peeled and halved medium ripe avocados
• 120 g mayonnaise
• 30 ml lemon juice
• 2 tins (170 g each) drained lump crabmeat
• 60 g fresh cilantro, chopped
• 30 g finely minced chives
• 1 seeded and minced serrano pepper
• 15 g drained capers
• 1 g pepper
• 250 g pepper jack cheese, shredded
• 2 g paprika
• slices of lemon

Directions:
• Pre-heat the broiler.
• In a large mixing basin, mash 2 avocado halves lightly with a fork.
• Mix in the mayonnaise and lemon juice until fully combined.
• Combine crab, 45 g cilantro, chives, serrano pepper, capers, and pepper in a mixing bowl.
• Fill the remaining avocado halves with the sauce.
• Place in a 15x10x1-inch baking pan.
• Garnish with paprika and cheese.
• Broil 4-5 inches from the heat for 3-5 minutes, or until the cheese is melted.
• Serve with the remaining cilantro and lemon wedges.

Nutrient value: 1 piece
• Calories: 325 kcal
• Carbohydrates: 6 g
• Protein: 14 g
• Fat: 28 g

Prep Time: 40 minutes
Cook Time: 0 minutes
Servings: 10 people

Ingredients:
• 450 g part-skim mozzarella cheese, cubed
• 24 florets of fresh broccoli (about 10 ounces)
• 120 g vinaigrette (Greek)
• 24 firm salami slices
• 2 jars (200 g each) delicious red peppers, roasted, drained, and sliced into 24 strips

Directions:
• Combine the cheese, broccoli, and vinaigrette in a shallow dish.
• Cover and refrigerate for 4 hours or overnight.
• Drain the cheese and broccoli while retaining the vinaigrette.
• Thread cheese, salami, broccoli, and peppers alternately on 24 appetiser skewers.
• Drizzle with the reserved vinaigrette.

Nutrient value: Per piece
• Calories: 109 kcal
• Carbohydrates: 2 g
• Protein: 9 g
• Fat: 7 g

Prep Time: 30 minutes
Cook Time: 0 minutes
Servings: 4 people

Ingredients:
• 450 g ground beef, lean (90 percent lean)
• 2 g of salt
• 1 g pepper
• 8 leaves Bibb lettuce
• 75 g feta cheese, crumbled
• 30 g of Miracle Whip Light
• 1/2 ripe medium avocado, peeled and cut into 8

slices
- 75 g red onion, chopped
- Optional: chopped cherry tomatoes

Directions:
- Combine beef, salt, and pepper in a large mixing basin, tossing lightly but thoroughly.
- Form into eight 1/2-inch thick patties.
- Grill the burgers, covered, over medium heat for 3-4 minutes on each side, or broil 3-4 inches from the heat until a thermometer reads 160°.
- Sandwich the patties between lettuce leaves.
- Spread feta and Miracle Whip on top of the burgers.
- Top with avocado, red onion, and tomatoes, if desired.

Nutrient value: 2 pieces
- Calories: 252 kcal
- Carbohydrates: 5 g
- Protein: 24 g
- Fat: 15 g

---

8. Chicken Tex-Mex Strips

Prep Time: 20minutes
Cook Time: 40 minutes
Servings: 4people

Ingredients:
- 120 g corn chips, finely crushed
- 60 g panko bread crumbs
- 15 g dry bread crumbs
- 60 g Mexican cheese blend, finely shredded
- 75 g taco seasoning
- a pinch of cayenne pepper
- 60 g melted butter
- 450 g tenderloins of chicken

Directions:
- Preheat the oven to 204ºC.
- Combine the first six ingredients in a small bowl.
- In a separate shallow bowl, place the butter.

- Dip the chicken in the butter, then roll it in the crumb mixture to coat and press to adhere. Place the chicken in a 15x10x1-inch baking tray lined with foil.
- Bake for 15 minutes, or until a thermometer inserted into the chicken reads 165°, rotating halfway through.

Nutrient value: Whole food
- Calories: 258 kcal
- Carbohydrates: 7 g
- Protein: 29 g
- Fat: 14 g

---

9. Guacamole With Cajun Shrimp And Red Pepper

Prep Time: 15 minutes
Cook Time: 5 minutes
Servings: 6 people

Ingredients:
- 3 peeled and cubed medium ripe avocados
- 45 ml fresh lime juice
- 5 g kosher salt
- Cajun Shrimp (220 g)
- 60 g sweet red pepper, chopped

Directions:
- Mash avocados in a mixing basin until almost smooth.
- Mix in the lime juice and 2 g salt.
- Allow flavours to mix for 10 minutes.
- If necessary, add more lime juice and salt to taste.
- Cajun Shrimp with red pepper flakes on top.

Nutrient value: Per serving
- Calories: 152 kcal
- Carbohydrates: 5 g
- Protein: 9 g
- Fat: 11 g

Prep Time: 15 minutes
Cook Time: 0 minutes
Servings: 12 people

Ingredients:
* 2 jars (200 g each) artichoke hearts marinated
* 30 ml vinegar (red wine)
* 30 ml olive oil
* 6 plum tomatoes, cut
* 450 g fresh mozzarella cheese, sliced
* 30 g fresh basil leaves, loosely packed
* Optional coarsely ground pepper

Directions:
* Drain the artichokes and set aside 120 g of the marinade.
* Whisk together the vinegar, oil, and reserved marinade in a small basin.
* Arrange the artichokes, tomatoes, mozzarella cheese, and basil on a large serving plate.
* Drizzle with vinaigrette and serve. Sprinkle with roughly ground pepper, if preferred.

Nutrient value: Per serving
* Calories: 192 kcal
* Carbohydrates: 4 g
* Protein: 8 g
* Fat: 16 g

Prep Time: 10minutes
Cook Time: 30 minutes
Servings: 4 people

Ingredients:
* 10 g dill (fresh)
* 3 g pepper
* 3 g salt
* 3 g powdered garlic
* Salmon fillets, 680 g

* 60 g brown sugar, packed
* 1 cube of chicken bouillon, combined with 45 ml water
* 45 ml of oil
* Soy sauce (45 ml)
* green onions, finely chopped (60 g)
* 2 slice onions, separated into rings 1 lemon, thinly sliced

Directions:
* Season the salmon with dill, pepper, salt, and garlic powder.
* Fill a shallow glass pan halfway with water.
* Combine the sugar, chicken broth, oil, soy sauce, and green onions in a mixing bowl.
* Pour the sauce over the salmon.
* Cover and chill for 1 hour, turning halfway through.
* Drain and toss out the marinade.
* Place lemon and onion on top of grill on medium heat.
* Cook for 15 minutes, or until the fish is cooked through.

Nutrient value:
* Calories: 380 kcal
* Carbohydrates: 170 g
* Protein: 37 g
* Fat: 17g

Prep Time: 15 minutes
Cook Time: 30 minutes
Servings: 2 people

Ingredients:
* 2 vine-ripened tomatoes, seeded and cut into 1/4-inch chunks
* 1 ripe avocado, peeled, pitted, and quartered
* 15 g red onion, chopped
* 10 g freshly squeezed lemon juice
* Tabasco sauce, 2 g

- a pinch of salt and pepper
- sour cream 60 g
- 45 g fresh coriander, chopped
- flour tortillas, 24 inch
- 3 ml oil (vegetable)
- 315 g monterey jack cheese, shredded

Directions:
- Combine the tomatoes, avocado, onion, lemon juice, and Tabasco in a small bowl.
- Season with salt and pepper to taste.
- Mix sour cream, coriander, salt, and pepper to taste in a separate small bowl.
- Brush the tops of the tortillas with oil and place them on a baking pan.
- 2 to 4 inches from the flame, broil tortillas until pale golden.
- Sprinkle cheese evenly over tortillas and broil until melted.
- To create 2 quesadillas, spread avocado mixture evenly over 2 tortillas and top each with 1 of the remaining tortillas, cheese side down.
- Cut the quesadillas into four wedges on a chopping board.
- Serve heated with a dollop of sour cream mixture on top of each wedge.

Nutrient value:
- Calories: 794 kcal
- Carbohydrates: 51 g
- Protein: 29 g
- Fat: 58 g

---

13. TACOS WITH VEGAN FRIED 'FISH'

Prep Time: 10 minutes
Cook Time: 40 minutes
Servings: 8 people

Ingredients:
- 475 g panko breadcrumbs
- 396 g silken tofu
- 120 g unbleached flour
- 2 g of salt
- smoked paprika 4 g
- cayenne pepper, 2 g
- 4 g cumin powder
- 120 ml vegetable oil (nondairy milk) for frying
- finely shredded head cabbage
- 1 avocado, ripe
- 8 tiny vegan mayonnaise tortillas to serve

ONION PICKLED
- 1 peeled and thinly sliced red onion
- Apple cider vinegar (60 ml)
- 15 g of sugar 4 g of salt

Directions:
- To remove excess moisture, pat the tofu with a few pieces of kitchen paper. Break the tofu into rough 1-inch chunks with a knife — I like them to be uneven, not cubes, so they look prettier!
- Put the breadcrumbs in a large shallow basin.
- In a separate large shallow basin, combine the flour, salt, smoked paprika, cayenne pepper, and cumin.
- Fill a third wide shallow basin halfway with milk.
- Toss the tofu chunks in the flour, then the milk, then the breadcrumbs, and place them on a baking sheet.
- Fill a deep frying pan halfway with vegetable oil.
- Place over a medium heat and allow the oil to heat up — if a breadcrumb begins to bubble and brown, the oil is ready.
- Fry chunks of breaded tofu in the oil till golden on the bottom, then flip and cook until golden all over.
- Drain on a baking sheet coated with kitchen paper.
- Repeat with the rest of the tofu.
- In a small saucepan, heat the apple cider vinegar, salt, and sugar until steaming.
- Pour the boiling vinegar over the thinly chopped red onion in a bowl or jar.
- Allow it to soften and spin for at least 30 minutes.

Nutrient value: Per Recipe
- Calories: 378 kcal
- Carbohydrates: 58 g

- Protein: 12g
- Fat: 10 g

Prep Time: 15 minutes
Cook Time: 20 minutes
Servings: 4 people

Ingredients:
- tilapia fillets, 900 g
- lemon juice (30 ml)
- 120 g parmesan cheese, grated
- 60 g room temperature butter
- mayonnaise (45 ml)
- 45 g green onions, finely chopped
- 1 g salt for seasoning
- 1 g dried basil, ground black pepper
- 1 g spicy pepper sauce

Directions:
- Preheat the oven to 176°C.
- Lay fillets in a single layer in a buttered 13-by-9-inch baking dish or jellyroll pan.
- Fillets should not be stacked.
- Brush the top with the juice.
- Combine the cheese, butter, mayonnaise, onions, and seasonings in a mixing bowl.
- Mix thoroughly with a fork.
- Bake the fish in a warm oven for 10 to 20 minutes, or until it begins to flake.
- Spread with the cheese mixture and bake for 5 minutes, or until golden brown.
- The baking time will be determined by the thickness of the fish used.
- Keep a tight eye on the fish to ensure it does not overcook.
- This recipe serves 4 people.
- It should be noted that this fish can also be prepared in a broiler.
- Broil for 3 to 4 minutes, or until nearly done.
- Broil for another 2 to 3 minutes, or until the cheese is browned.

Nutrient value: Per Serving
- Calories: 376 kcal
- Carbohydrates: 1 g
- Protein: 50 g
- Fat: 12 g

Prep Time: 15 minutes
Cook Time: 15 minutes
Servings: 6 people

Ingredients:
- 2 bacon pieces
- 1 finely sliced small yellow onion
- 1 g of salt (or to taste)
- 60 ml of water
- 15 g Dijon mustard
- 450 g Brussels sprouts, trimmed, halved, and thinly sliced
- 15 ml cider vinegar

Directions:
- In a large skillet over medium heat, cook bacon until crisp (5 to 7 minutes); drain on paper towels, then crumble.
- Add the onion and salt to the pan drippings and cook over medium heat, turning frequently, until soft and browned (about 3 minutes).
- Scrape up any browned pieces with the water and mustard, then add the Brussels sprouts and simmer, stirring frequently, until soft (4 to 6 minutes).
- Stir in the vinegar and sprinkle with the crumbled bacon.

Nutrient value: Per serving
- Calories: 45 kcal
- Carbohydrates: 5 g
- Protein: 3 g
- Fat: 14 g

16. Popcorn Roasted Cauliflower

Prep Time: 5 minutes
Cook Time: 1 hour
Servings: 4 people

Ingredients:
- 1 head cauliflower or 1 head similar amount of commercially prepared pre-cut cauliflower
- 60 ml olive oil
- 2 g salt (adjusted to taste)

Directions:
- Preheat the oven to 218°C.
- Remove the core and thick stems from the cauliflower head; cut the florets into ping-pong-sized pieces.
- In a large mixing bowl, whisk together the olive oil and salt, then add the cauliflower pieces and toss thoroughly.
- Line a baking sheet with parchment paper for easy cleanup (if you don't have any), then spread the cauliflower pieces on the sheet and roast for 1 hour, turning 3 or 4 times, until most of each piece has gone golden brown.
- (The more caramelization that occurs and the sweeter the cauliflower pieces taste, the browner they get.)
- Serve right away and enjoy!

Nutrient value: Per recipe
- Calories: 156 kcal
- Carbohydrates: 6 g
- Protein: 3 g
- Fat: 13 g

---

17 Best Baked Potato

Prep Time: 10 minutes
Cook Time: 1 hour
Servings: 2 people

Ingredients:
- 1 big russet potato
- 15 ml canola oil
- kosher salt

Directions:
- Preheat the oven to 176°C and place racks in the top and bottom thirds.
- Wash the potato (or potatoes) thoroughly under cold running water with a vigorous brush.
- Allow to dry before poking 8 to 12 deep holes all over the spud with a regular fork to allow moisture to escape during cooking.
- Place in a bowl and lightly coat with oil.
- Sprinkle with kosher salt and set potato on a rack in the centre of the oven.
- To collect any drippings, place a baking sheet (I used aluminium foil) on the bottom rack.
- Bake for 1 hour, or until the skin is crisp but the flesh beneath is tender.
- Create a dotted line from end to end with your fork, then crack the potato open by squeezing the ends together.
- It will pop right open.
- But watch out, there will be some steam.

Nutrient value: Per recipe
- Calories: 284 kcal
- Carbohydrates: 30 g
- Protein: 20 g
- Fat: 1 g

---

18. Lentil Burgers

Prep Time: 10 minutes
Cook Time: 1 hour
Servings: 5 people

Ingredients:
- 250 g well-rinsed dried lentils
- 600 ml water
- 2 g salt
- 15 ml olive oil
- 12 medium diced onion

- 1 diced carrot
- 2 g black pepper
- 5 ml soy sauce
- 60 g finely milled rolled oats
- 75 g breadcrumbs

Directions:
- Cook lentils in salted water for about 45 minutes.
- The lentils will be mushy and most of the water will have evaporated.
- Fry the onions and carrot in the oil for about 5 minutes, or until tender.
- Combine the cooked ingredients with the pepper, soy sauce, oats, and bread cumbs in a mixing bowl.
- Form the ingredients into patties while it is still heated; this will yield 8-10 burgers.
- Burgers can then be shallow fried for 1-2 minutes on each side or baked for 15 minutes at 200 degrees Celsius.

Nutrient value: Per piece
- Calories: 176 kcal
- Carbohydrates: 3 g
- Protein: 9 g
- Fat: 3 g

19. Muffins With Coconut Kefir And Banana

Prep Time: 10 minutes
Cook Time: 30 minutes
Servings: 10 people

Ingredients:
- 450 g AP flour
- 250 g sugar, granulated
- 250 g dried shredded unsweetened coconut
- 10 g baking powder
- 3 g baking powder
- 2 g of salt
- mashed 2 ripe bananas
- 120 g kefir probiotic fermented coconut milk (dairy-free)
- 100 ml liquid cold-pressed coconut oil

- 5 ml vanilla extract

Directions:
- Preheat the oven to 180ºC. Cooking spray should be sprayed into a 12-count muffin tray. Place aside.
- In a large mixing basin, combine the flour, sugar, coconut, baking soda, baking powder, and salt. Place aside.
- In a separate big mixing basin, combine the bananas, kefir, coconut oil, and vanilla. Stir in until no white streaks remain in the flour mixture.
- Divide the batter evenly into the prepared muffin tin wells. Bake for 30 minutes, or until the tops are golden and a toothpick inserted into the centers comes out clean. Allow to cool in the muffin tray for 15 minutes.

Nutrient value: Per Piece
- Calories: 300kcal
- Carbohydrates: 12 g
- Protein: 4 g
- Fat: 15 g

20. Crisp Berry

Prep Time: 10 minutes
Cook Time: 30 minutes
Servings: 6 people

Ingredients:

FRUIT
- 450 g bag cherries or 450 g bag blueberries
- 100 g box jello sugar-free vanilla pudding mix, cooked and served
- 15 g cinnamon
- 3 g ground nutmeg
- 75 ml fat-free milk

CRISP
- 120 g old fashioned oats
- 120 g Splenda (or other sugar substitute)

- 220 g fat-free plain yoghurt
- 5 ml almond extract

Directions:
- Coat an 8X8 baking pan with cooking spray.
- In the pan, combine the fruit components and mix well.
- Crisp mix should be combined in a separate bowl.
- To construct a top crust, spread this mixture over the berry mixture.
- Bake for 40-45 minutes, or until the topping becomes crunchy, at 176°C.

Nutrient value: Per serving
- Calories: 121 kcal
- Carbohydrates: 7 g
- Protein: 4 g
- Fat: 2 g

CHAPTER 15

RECIPES PASTA

1. PASTA WITH CREAMY SALMON

Prep Time: 5 minutes
Cook Time: 15 minutes
Servings: 3 people

Ingredients:
- 170 g farfalle
- 30 g melted butter
- Salmon, 200 g.
- 2 garlic cloves
- 10 g all-purpose flour
- 100 ml white wine, dry
- 100 ml chicken stock (or vegetable stock)
- 120 g heavy cream chives - for decoration
- fresh ground black pepper and fine sea salt

Directions:
- To prepare the salmon:
- Preheat a nonstick ceramic skillet to a temperature just below medium.
- Melt the butter in the skillet.
- Season the salmon generously with sea salt and freshly ground pepper and place it in the pan.
- Cook for 5 minutes on the first side, then flip and cook for another 3-5 minutes, depending on the thickness of the fish.
- Remove the salmon from the pan and season with salt and pepper. Sautee for a few minutes, then toss in the flour.
- To prepare the sauce:
- Add the wine to the pan and scrape everything ad-hered to the bottom of the pan into the liquid with a wooden spoon.
- Allow the wine to come to a boil while constantly stirring to ensure there are no lumps in the sauce.
- Allow the sauce to barely begin to boil before reducing to a low heat with the stock and cream.
- Allow the sauce to thicken for a few minutes on low heat.
- The pasta should have completed cooking as the sauce thickens.
- Set aside after draining.
- When the sauce has thickened, add the farfalle to the skillet and stir to coat.
- Break the salmon into small chunks with a fork or knife and add to the spaghetti, stirring to combine.
- Garnish with chives and serve.

Nutrient value: Whole recipe
- Calories: 840 kcal
- Carbohydrates: 50 g
- Protein: 29g
- Fat: 45 g

---

2. SQUASH CASSEROLE WITH CHICKEN SPAGHETTI

Prep Time: 25 minutes
Cook Time: 20 minutes
Servings: 8 people

Ingredients:

- 1 spaghetti squash, medium
- 75 g butter
- 1 kg cooked shredded chicken
- 250 g celery, diced
- 1 medium onion, diced
- 1 diced poblano pepper
- 1 diced bell pepper
- 5 garlic cloves minced garlic
- 100 ml chicken broth
- 250 g diced can drained chilis and tomatoes (like Ratel)
- 1 kg thick cream
- 120 g cream cheese
- 3 g garlic powder
- 2 g cumin
- 1 g pepper
- 350g Colby Jack cheese, shredded

Directions:

- Preheat the oven to 220°C.
- Microwave the squash whole for 4-5 minutes to soften it before cutting.
- When removing, use caution because the skin will be heated.
- Trim both ends of the squash and cut lengthwise down the centre to create two boats.
- Scrape and scrape out the seeds, then throw them away.
- Drizzle olive oil over the sliced side of the squash and season with salt.
- Place the cut side down on a parchment-lined sheet pan and roast for 30 minutes, or until cooked.
- While the squash is baking, heat the butter in a big skillet.
- Cook for about 7 minutes, or until the onion, bell pepper, celery, and poblano are softened, over medium high heat.
- Cook for another 1-2 minutes after adding the garlic.
- Combine the chicken stock, tomatoes, and chilis in a mixing bowl.
- and continue to boil until the stock has been reduced by half.
- There should be roughly 45 ml of liquid remaining.
- Add the cream to the vegetables and cook until it is reduced and thickened. Remove from the heat and transfer the veggie mixture to a large mixing bowl.
- Combine cream cheese, salt, pepper, garlic, and cumin in a mixing bowl.
- Stir until everything is mixed and the cream cheese is melted.
- After 30 minutes, carefully take the squash from the oven and flip it over.
- The squash should be soft on top but not fully cooked through.
- Remove the spaghetti squash from the peel using a fork.
- If there is excess moisture from the cooked squash, place it on some paper towels to absorb the moisture.
- Reduce the oven temperature to 176°C.
- Mix the squash into the veggie mixture gently.
- Then, gently fold in 120 g cheese and the chicken.
- Fill a greased casserole dish or 913 pan halfway with the squash and chicken mixture.
- Bake for 20 minutes, or until warmed through and the cheese is melted and bubbling, at 176°C.
- Allow for a 10-minute rest before diving in!

Nutrient value: Per serving

- Calories: 466 kcal
- Carbohydrates: 5 g
- Protein: 25 g
- Fat: 37 g

---

3. KETO LASAGNA

Prep Time: 5 minutes
Cook Time: 10 minutes
Servings: 4 people

Ingredients:

- 450 g sausage (ground)
- Marinara sauce made with low-carb ingredients (you can also use sugar-free pizza sauce)

- 250 g of shredded mozzarella cheese
- 250 g of ricotta cheese (you can also use cottage cheese)
- 250 g Parmesan cheese
- 75 g garlic
- 2 g Italian spice
- 1 g teaspoon salt
- 1 g pepper

Directions:
- Preheat the oven to 190°C.
- Brown the sausage in a skillet.
- Combine the parmesan cheese, ricotta, garlic powder, Italian seasoning, and salt in a mixing bowl.
- Lasagna in a Bowl on a Keto Diet
- Fill your bowls with 1/4 of the sausage, 1/4 of the sauce, 1/4 of the ricotta, and roughly 1/4 (or more if preferred) of the shredded mozzarella cheese.
- Lasagna in a Bowl on a Keto Diet
- Place the bowls on a sheet pan and bake until the cheese is melted (approximately 10 minutes), or microwave for about 3-5 minutes until the cheese is melted.

Nutrient value: Per serving
- Calories: 130 kcal
- Carbohydrates: 1 g
- Protein: 2 g
- Fat: 5

---

4. KETO MUSHROOM PASTA

Prep Time: 20 minutes
Cook Time: 40 minutes
Servings: 4 people

Ingredients:
- 1 package Palmini palm hearts linguini
- 450 ml choice of milk
- 45 g unsalted butter
- 170 g sliced mushrooms
- 450 g fresh baby spinach
- 220 g riced cauliflower
- 250 g vegetable stock, garlic powder
- shredded parmesan cheese, seasoned with salt and pepper (optional)

Directions:
- Heat 30 g butter in a large stovetop pan.
- Season the riced cauliflower with salt, pepper, and garlic powder.
- Cook, stirring often, over medium heat until translucent/slightly brown (about 6-8 minutes).
- Cool for a few minutes.
- Drain the Palmini pasta and thoroughly rinse it with water.
- Transfer to a bowl and soak for 15-30 minutes in milk.
- Place aside.
- Combine the cooked cauliflower and 120 g vegetable stock in a blender or food processor.
- Blend until smooth, adding more liquid if necessary.
- 15 g butter, heated in a separate pan on the stovetop
- Cook the mushrooms for 6-7 minutes over medium heat, or until softened/cooked through.
- Stir in the spinach until it begins to wilt.
- Reduce the heat to low.
- Drain and rinse the pasta once more, then add it to the pan with the spinach and mushroom mixture, followed by roughly 250 g of the cauliflower cream sauce (keep the remainder for something else!).
- Mix everything together and cook for about 5 minutes on low heat, or until the pasta achieves the desired softened consistency.
- Garnish with parmesan cheese.

Nutrient value: Per serving
- Calories: 230 kcal
- Carbohydrates: 10 g
- Protein: 29 g
- Fat: 25 g

Prep Time: 5 minutes
Cook Time: 12 minutes
Servings: 4 people

Ingredients:
- 6 slices bacon
- 30 ml extra-virgin olive oil
- 2 minced garlic cloves
- 1 diced tomato
- 1 kg zoodles
- 120 g blue cheese crumbles
- 2 cut basil leaves

Directions:
- Cook bacon in a large skillet over medium-high heat until crisp. Place aside. When completely cool, cut into crumbles.
- Remove everything except one tablespoon of bacon fat from the skillet.
- Heat the olive oil and garlic cloves over medium heat.
- Cook for 1 minute, or until aromatic.
- Mix in the tomatoes.
- Cook until the diced tomatoes are softened, about 3 minutes.
- Cook for 2 minutes, or until the sauce has incorperated over the zoodles and the zucchini noodles are heated through but still firm to the touch.
- Turn off the heat and stir in the blue cheese crumbles and basil.
- Season with salt and pepper to taste.
- Serve right away.

Nutrient value: Per serving
- Calories: 260 kcal
- Carbohydrates: 4 g
- Protein: 14 g
- Fat: 19 g

Prep Time: 20 minutes
Cook Time: 45 minutes
Servings: 8 people

Ingredients:
- 1 courgette
- 10 ml olive oil
- 450 g minced beef
- 3 g salt and 2 g pepper
- 3 g of Italian seasoning
- 1 g anise seeds
- 350 ml low carb marinara sauce
- 75 g ricotta cheese
- 75 g parmesan cheese, grated
- ONE EGG
- 3 g garlic powder
- 250 g sliced fresh mozzarella cheese

Directions:
- Preheat the oven to 202°C.
- Remove the zucchini's ends and set aside.
- Cut the zucchini into thin strips lengthwise with a mandoline slicer.
- Place the zucchini on a plate or chopping board and sprinkle with a very thin layer of salt.
- Allow for a 15-minute resting period.
- After that, blot the zucchini to remove any excess moisture.
- While the zucchini is drying, heat the olive oil in a skillet over medium heat. Cook for 2-3 minutes after adding the ground beef.
- Season with salt, pepper, Italian seasoning, and anise seeds to taste.
- Cook until the ground meat is cooked through.
- Add 250 g marinara sauce.
- Simmer for around 1-2 minutes.
- Take the pan off the heat and set it aside.
- Make the white sauce while the ground beef is cooking.
- In a small bowl, combine ricotta, egg, parmesan and
- Make the lasagna.

- Fill a small casserole dish halfway with 120 g marinara sauce.
- Create a layer of zucchini noodles.
- Half of the ground beef mixture should be on top.
- Half of the white sauce should be spread on top.
- Half of the mozzarella cheese should be layered on the bottom.
- Layers should be repeated.
- Bake at 400 degrees Fahrenheit for 25 to 30 minutes.
- Allow to cool for 3-5 minutes before serving.

Nutrient value: Per serving
- Calories: 333 kcal
- Carbohydrates: 2 g
- Protein: 13 g
- Fat: 25 g

7. Creamy Keto Pumpkin Alfredo

Prep Time: 10 minutes
Cook Time: 20 minutes
Servings: 6 people

Ingredients:
- 30 g melted butter
- 2 minced garlic cloves
- 250 g pureed pumpkin
- 1kg thick cream
- 1 g black pepper
- 2 g salt
- 1 g ground nutmeg
- 120 g parmesan cheese, shredded
- 1.5 kg zoodles

Directions:
- Melt butter in a large skillet over medium heat. Then add the garlic and simmer for 1 minute, or until the garlic is aromatic.
- Pour in the pumpkin and whisk to mix.
- Combine heavy cream, salt, pepper, and nutmeg in a mixing bowl. Simmer over medium heat for 3-5 mi-

nutes, or until the sauce has thickened.
- Remove from the heat once the sauce has thickened and stir in the parmesan cheese. Serve with the zucchini noodles.

Nutrient value: Per serving
- Calories: 218 kcal
- Carbohydrates: 6 g
- Protein: 5 g
- Fat: 8 g

8. Alfredo Creamy Keto Garlic And Olive Pasta

Prep Time: 5 minutes
Cook Time: 15 minutes
Servings: 6 people

Ingredients:
- 10 g melted butter
- 2 minced garlic cloves
- 1.5 Kg thick cream
- 1 yolk of an egg
- 250 g grated parmesan cheese
- 250 g chopped green olives
- Salt & pepper to taste
- 1.5 kg zoodles

Directions:
- Melt butter in a large skillet over medium heat.
- Then add the garlic and simmer for 1 minute, or until the garlic is aromatic.
- Whisk together the cream and egg yolk in a small mixing bowl until incorporated.
- Pour the cream mixture into the skillet with the garlic butter one tablespoon at a time.
- Stir until everything is mixed.
- Cook, stirring constantly, until the mixture thickens.
- Approximately 5-7 minutes.
- Remove the sauce from the heat after it has thickened.
- Stir in the green olives, parmesan cheese, and sea-

son with salt and pepper to suit.
- Mix in the zucchini noodles.
- Allow to sit for 2-3 minutes, or until the zoodles soften.

Nutrient value: Per serving
- Calories: 385 kcal
- Carbohydrates: 7 g
- Protein: 7 g
- Fat: 37 g

---

9. Keto Feta Baked Pasta

Prep Time: 20minutes
Cook Time: 35 minutes
Servings: 4 people

Ingredients:
- 2 kg grape tomatoes
- 2 minced garlic cloves
- 120 ml extra-virgin olive oil
- feta cheese, 200 g solid block
- three basil leaves
- 450 g Kalamata olives
- 250 g chicken shredded
- 3 g sea salt
- 190 g hearts of palm or zucchini noodles

Directions:
- Preheat the oven to 202°C.
- Fill a large casserole dish halfway with tomatoes. Sprinkle with garlic powder.
- To the tomatoes and garlic, add the olive oil. Toss to coat evenly.
- In the centre of the casserole dish, place a block of feta cheese. Bake at 202°C for 30–45 minutes, or until the feta is creamy.
- Stir in the basil, olives, chicken, salt, and noodles after removing from the oven.

Nutrient value: Per serving
- Calories: 343 kcal
- Carbohydrates: 3 g
- Protein: 14g
- Fat: 26 g

---

10. Chicken And Asparagus "Pasta" With Creamy Avocado

Prep Time: 2 minutes
Cook Time: 10 minutes
Servings: 2 people

Ingredients:
- 4 medium spiralized zucchinis
- 350 g boneless, skinless chicken breast, split into strips
- 1 g Himalayan salt
- 1 g freshly ground black pepper
- 1 big shredded endive
- 12 spears fresh asparagus, sliced into 2-3 inch pieces
- 75 g chopped walnuts
- 30 g chopped fresh parsley

For the avocado cream sauce
- 1 avocado, large and ripe
- 120 ml unsweetened coconut milk
- 1 lemon's juice
- 120 ml water
- 3 g Himalayan salt
- 1 g freshly ground black pepper
- 3 g fresh thyme

Directions:
- Set aside your zucchini noodles in a large mixing basin after spiralizing them using a spiralizer.
- In a medium skillet over medium-high heat, melt a little amount of cooking butter and add the chicken.
- Season with salt and pepper and simmer for 5-6 minutes, or until thoroughly cooked.
- Continue cooking the endive and asparagus for 3-4 minutes, or until the vegetables are soft.
- While the chicken and vegetables are cooking, combine all of the avocado sauce ingredients in a mini

food processor and puree until smooth and creamy.
- Mix the reserved zucchinis with the chicken and vegetables.
- The heat from this will be enough to "cook" the zucchinis and soften them.
- Mix in the avocado.
- Mix and serve

Nutrient value: Whole recipe
- Calories: 636 kcal
- Carbohydrates: 30 g
- Protein: 53 g
- Fat: 36 g

---

11. Noodles With Zucchini

Prep Time: 10 minutes
Cook Time: 6 hours
Servings: 6 people

Ingredients:
To make the sauce
- 800 g organic tomato puree
- organic 175 g can tomato paste
- 120 g chicken stock
- 15 ml olive oil
- 10 g Italian herb blend
- 3 g kosher salt
- 3 g pepper
- 1 g crushed red pepper flakes
- 3 minced garlic cloves
- 2 sliced tiny carrots
- 1 small sliced onion
- 450 g turkey ground

To make zucchini noodles
3–6 medium zucchini

Directions:
To prepare sauce
- Stir together all of the sauce ingredients except the turkey in the slow cooker.
- Cut the ground turkey into cubes and place it in the slow cooker with the sauce.
- Stirring is not permitted.
- Cook for 6-8 hours on low heat.
- When the sauce is finished, break up the ground turkey into small chunks with a potato masher.
- **In order to create zucchini noodles,** Spiralize 12 - 1 medium zucchini per serving.
- In a large frying pan, heat 1 tablespoon olive oil over medium heat.
- Cook zucchini for 3 minutes, or until warmed through but still firm.

Nutrient value: Whole recipe
- Calories: 231 kcal
- Carbohydrates: 27 g
- Protein: 28 g
- Fat: 5 g

---

12. Shrimp Roasted In Garlic With Zucchini Pasta

Prep Time: 10 minutes
Cook Time: 10 minutes
Servings: 2 people

Ingredients:
- 250 g peeled and deveined frozen shrimp
- 10 ml olive oil
- 10 g melted ghee (or additional olive oil)
- 2 minced garlic cloves
- 1 g salt fresh ground pepper to taste
- 1 lemon, zested and juiced
- 2 zucchini (medium)

Directions:
- Preheat the oven to 202°C.
- In a baking dish, combine the shrimp, olive oil, ghee, garlic, lemon zest, lemon juice, salt, and pepper.
- Toss to coat the shrimp.
- Bake for 8-10 minutes, rotating halfway through.
- Cook until the shrimp are pink and almost done, or until heated through if using pre-cooked shrimp.

- Toss in the zucchini spaghetti and serve.

Nutrient value:
Per serving
- Calories: 409 kcal
- Carbohydrates: 8 g
- Protein: 25 g
- Fat: 31 g

---

13. Pesto Zucchini Pasta

Prep Time: 25 minutes
Cook Time: 5 minutes
Servings: 4 people

Ingredients:
- 2 big zucchini seasoned with salt
- 250 g sliced cherry tomatoes
- **To make the pesto**
- 100 g toasted walnuts
- 1 roasted garlic head
- 450 g fresh basil leaves, plus a couple for garnish
- 5 ml lemon juice
- 75 ml extra virgin olive oil

Directions:
- To create zucchini noodles, spiralize or julienne the zucchini.
- Lightly salt zucchini and drain for 20 minutes in a strainer to remove excess liquid.
- Toast the walnuts in an oven at 276°C for 8-10 minutes, or until lightly browned and fragrant.
- Allow to cool to room temperature before serving.
- In a food processor, combine roasted garlic cloves, cooled walnuts, and a generous amount of sea salt.
- Pulse the mixture until it resembles large crumbs.
- Combine the basil leaves and lemon juice in a mixing bowl.
- While the processor is running, drizzle in the olive oil.
- Scrape down the bowl's sides and process until barely blended.

- To taste, add more sea salt.
- Toss the drained zucchini noodles and tomatoes with the pesto in a large mixing bowl until fully incorporated.
- Garnish with fresh basil if desired.

Nutrient value:
Per serving
- Calories: 220 kcal
- Carbohydrates: 9 g
- Protein: 4 g
- Fat: 20 g

---

14. Zoodles Of Easy Chicken Veggie Stir Fry

Prep Time: 10 minutes
Cook Time: 15 minutes
Servings: 4 people

Ingredients:
Marinade for chicken
- 450 g boneless and skinless chicken thighs
- 15 ml toasted sesame oil plus more for stir-frying
- 15 ml extra virgin organic olive oil
- 2 minced garlic cloves
- 2 g sea salt
- 2 g fresh grated ginger
- 1 g red pepper flakes

Stir-Fry Veggies
- four huge zucchini
- 5 cut green onions, including whites and some green bits
- 450 g florets fresh broccoli
- 2 carrots, sliced into thin matchsticks
- 175 g snow or snap peas
- 1 red pepper, cut into strips
- 450 g cremini mushrooms, sliced
- 100 g of coconut aminos
- 2 g fresh grated ginger
- 1 garlic clove, minced,
- Sea salt to taste

Directions:
- Trim any excess fat from the chicken and cut it into one-inch pieces.
- In a medium mixing basin, combine the chicken marinade ingredients.
- To coat the chicken evenly, toss it in the dressing.
- Place aside.
- Set aside zucchini noodles made with a spiralizer (or julienne peeler). (For further instructions on how to make zucchini noodles, see How to Spiralize in 3 Easy Steps.)
- Cut and slice the remaining vegetables as directed above, keeping the red pepper and mushrooms separate from the other ingredients.
- Then, in a wok or big sauté pan, heat the oil over medium-high heat.
- Add 1 tablespoon of toasted sesame oil to the pan once it's hot.
- Sauté the diced green onions for a minute or two, or until aromatic.
- Then, add the chicken, making care to distribute it evenly across the pan. Allow about a minute for the chicken to sear. Then, carefully toss the chicken to cook all sides until it is opaque (about 2 minutes).
- Combine the broccoli, carrots, and snow peas in a large mixing bowl. To blend, toss everything together thoroughly. Cook for around 2 minutes. Then stir in the coconut aminos, ginger, and garlic. Toss well to distribute equally throughout the veggie mixture. Cover pan for about 2 minutes, or until vegetables soften somewhat.
- Add the red pepper and mushrooms next. Toss well to combine ingredients and cook for 2 minutes, uncovered.
- Finally, throw in the zucchini noodles to mix. Cover the pan and steam cook the zucchini noodles until they reach the desired consistency. (We like ours better.)

Nutrient value: Per serving
- Calories: 322 kcal
- Carbohydrates: 25 g
- Protein: 29 g
- Fat: 13 g

15. SPAGHETTI SQUASH

Prep Time: 3 minutes
Cook Time: 12 minutes
Servings: 8 people

Ingredients:
- 1 medium spaghetti squash
- 250 ml water

Directions:
- In the cooking pot, place a steamer rack or trivet.
- Place the spaghetti squash on the rack and cover with water.
- Select Manual or Pressure Cook as the cooking mode.
- Set the pressure to high and the cook time to 12 minutes.
- Start the programme.
- When the cooking is finished, wait for the pressure to release (natural release).
- Remove the squash from the pot by lifting it out with the trivet handles. Place the squash on a cutting board and use tongs to split it in half. Remove the seeds and separate the strands with a fork.

Nutrient value: Per serving
- Calories: 33 kcal
- Carbohydrates: 5 g
- Protein: 0 g
- Fat: 0 g

16. SPAGHETTI WITH MEATBALLS (LOW CARB SPAGHETTI)

Prep Time: 10 minutes
Cook Time: 30 minutes
Servings: 4 people

Ingredients:
- 450 g minced beef
- 100 g almond flour, superfine
- 10 g Italian herb mixture
- 3 g dried oregano

- 3 g garlic powder
- 2 g of sea salt
- 1 EGG
- 15 g keto marina sauce

Directions:
- Preheat the oven to 176°C and spray an 8-inch cast iron pan or baking dish with avocado oil spray.
- In a large mixing bowl, combine the egg, almond flour, herbs, and spices.
- Add in the ground beef.
- Scoop, gently shape, and place meatballs in pan.
- 15 minutes in the oven
- Remove the meatballs from the oven and serve with marinara sauce.
- Return to the oven and cook for another 15 minutes, or until the internal temperature reaches 71°C and the sauce is simmering.

Nutrient value: Per serving
- Calories: 379 kcal
- Carbohydrates: 10g
- Protein: 20 g
- Fat: 24 g

---

17. NOODLES WITH CURRY BUTTERNUT SQUASH

Prep Time: 15 minutes
Cook Time: 15 minutes
Servings: 6 people

Ingredients:
- 30 ml avocado oil, split
- 1/2 inch peeled and grated fresh ginger
- 2 minced garlic cloves pinch red pepper flakes
- 15 g curry paste (green)
- 15 g green curry paste
- 2 g cumin
- 450 ml coconut milk (full fat)
- 10 ml lime juice, plus more to taste
- 5 ml fish sauce
- 3 g coconut sugar

- 2 g sea salt, plus more as desired
- 1 finely sliced yellow onion
- 1 thinly sliced red pepper
- 1 thinly sliced green pepper
- 700 g "noodles" made from butternut squash
- 250 g spinach, fresh (optional)
- 15 g finely sliced scallions

For Garnish
- 15 g cilantro
- 1 lime, peeled and split into wedges for garnish
- 1 red chile pepper, thinly sliced for garnish
- Optional: 250 g spinach, fresh

Directions:
Make the curry broth as follows:
- In a medium pot over medium-high heat, heat 15 ml oil.
- When the mixture is heated, add the ginger, garlic, red pepper flakes, green curry paste, and cumin. Cook for 1 minute, stirring occasionally.
- Combine the coconut milk, lime juice, fish sauce, coconut sugar, and sea salt in a mixing bowl.
- To blend, whisk everything together.
- Bring the sauce to a boil, then reduce to a low heat and leave to simmer for 10-15 minutes.
- Season with salt and pepper to taste.
- Meanwhile, sauté the following vegetables:
- In a large sauté pan, heat 15 ml oil.
- Add the peppers, onions, and a bit of salt and cook until the onions are translucent and the peppers begin to soften, about 3-5 minutes.
- Sauté the butternut squash "noodles" for an additional 5-7 minutes.
- If using spinach, add it at the end and toss until wilted.
- Divide the vegetables into serving bowls and top with the curry sauce.
- Garnish with cilantro, scallions, and, if using, red chile pepper, and serve immediately.

Nutrient value: Per serving
- Calories: 229 kcal
- Carbohydrates: 10 g

- Protein: 2 g
- Fat: 17 g

Prep Time: 5 minutes
Cook Time: 10 minutes
Servings: 3 people

Ingredients:

- 3 ml oil, avocado, coconut, or olive oil would suffice.
- 30 g minced red onion
- 1-2 rutabagas, peeled (should make about 3 cups of noodles)
- 100 ml unsweetened Almond Breeze almond milk
- 30 g pesto, freshly prepared
- To taste, 100 g grape tomatoes, diced smashed red pepper

Directions:

- To make rutabaga noodles, use a spiralizer.
- In a large skillet over medium-high heat, heat the oil.
- Sauté the onion for around 2 minutes.
- Cook for 2 minutes more after adding the spiralized rutabaga noodles to the skillet.
- Cook for 2-4 minutes more, or until the noodles have softened but still have a little firmness, after adding the almond milk.
- Stir in the pesto until well combined.
- Mix in the tomatoes and crushed red pepper.
- Serve immediately after removing from the heat.
- Any leftovers should be refrigerated.
- They can be eaten cold or reheated before serving.

Nutrient value: Per serving

- Calories: 167 kcal
- Carbohydrates: 10g
- Protein: 4 g
- Fat: 9 g

Prep Time: 10 minutes
Cook Time: 10 minutes
Servings: 4 people

Ingredients:

- 450 g asparagus, cut into noodles
- 15 g melted butter
- 1 kg thick cream
- 30 ml lemon juice and 3 ml lemon zest
- 3 g Dijon mustard
- 2 smashed garlic cloves
- 30 g grated Parmesan cheese

Directions:

- Begin with preparing the asparagus noodles.
- First, remove the tops and store them for later use or to add to this dish if desired.
- Hold the aparagus by the woody end and form ribbon noodles with a vegetable peeler.
- You should only have the woody stem and a portion of the spear left.
- In a small sauce pan, combine the cream, mustard, lemon juice, zest, and garlic.
- Bring it to a simmer with a whisk.
- After 5 minutes, add the parmesan cheese.
- Whisk one more until the cheese is melted and properly combined.
- Microwave the asparagus noodles for about 2 minutes during the allotted time.
- I prefer mine al dente, but if you prefer them softer, cook for an additional minute.

Nutrient value:

- Calories: 169 kcal
- Carbohydrates: 0g
- Protein: 2.9g
- Fat: 5g

Prep Time: 5 minutes

Cook Time: 20 minutes
Servings: 5 people

Ingredients:
- 225 g raw peeled and deveined shrimp
- 1 Asparagus bunch
- 225 g sliced Baby Bella or White Mushrooms
- 15 ml olive oil,
- salt, and pepper
- 1 medium spiralized celeriac
- 15 ml olive oil
- 1 smashed garlic clove
- 15 ml dried oregano
- 3 g Chili Flakes
- 3 ml Lemon Zest
- 5 ml Lemon Juice
- Walnuts,100 g

Directions:
- Preheat the oven to 202ºC.
- Place the shrimp, asparagus, and mushrooms on a baking sheet, drizzle with olive oil, and season with salt and pepper to taste.
- Place the skillet in the oven for 10 to 12 minutes, or until the shrimp are pink and opaque.
- While the shrimp is cooking, heat a tablespoon of olive oil in a large skillet over medium heat.
- Allow the crushed garlic, oregano, and chile to boil in the oil for about 2 minutes, taking care not to burn the garlic.
- Toss the celeriac noodles with the oil to coat.
- Cook for 4-5 minutes, depending on the size of the celeriac. Remove from the heat and place the noodles in a large mixing bowl. Combine the shrimp, asparagus, and mushrooms in a mixing bowl.
- Divide the mixture between two bowls and top with fresh lemon juice.
- Serve with the zest and walnuts, and enjoy!

Nutrient value: Per serving
- Calories: 130kcal
- Carbohydrates: 6 g
- Protein: 9 g
- Fat: 5 g

CHAPTER 16

RECIPES SOUPS AND STEWS

1. Miso Soup With Tofu And Greens

Prep Time: 5 minutes
Cook Time: 10 minutes
Servings: 4 people

Ingredients:
- 1.5 L vegetable stock
- 2 nori sheets
- 100 g miso paste (white or yellow)
- 250 g chopped green chard (or other tough green)
- 250 g green onion, chopped
- 120 g tofu (firm)

Directions:
- In a medium sauce pan, bring vegetable broth to a low simmer.
- Meanwhile, place miso (beginning at the low end of the range) in a small bowl, add a little boiling water, and whisk until smooth.
- This will prevent it from clumping when added to the soup later.
- Place aside.
- Cook for 5 minutes after adding the chard (or other greens of choice), green onion, and tofu (if using silken, add at the end of cooking) to the broth.
- Then stir in the nori. Remove from the heat and toss in the miso mixture.
- If desired, add extra miso or a pinch of sea salt.
- Serve hot. When it's fresh, it's best.

Nutrient value: Per serving
- Calories: 170 kcal
- Carbohydrates: 22 g
- Protein: 13 g
- Fat: 15 g

2. Thai Lemongrass Soup

Prep Time: 10 minutes
Cook Time: 15 minutes
Servings: 4 people

Ingredients:
- 2 lemongrass stalks (4 to 6 inches)
- 15 ml vegetable oil (divided)
- 2 minced garlic cloves
- 3 g ginger, freshly grated
- 3 g sambal oelek (or to taste)
- 1 L vegetable broth
- 450 g shiitake mushrooms, stemmed and sliced
- 250 g halved cherry tomatoes,
- 250 g extra firm tofu,
- 60 g chopped fresh cilantro
- 3 g lime juice
- Tamari or soy sauce

Directions:
- Bruise the lemongrass stalks by pressing them down with a large knife until they flatten slightly.
- Each stalk should be cut into four parts. Place

aside.
- In a medium saucepan, heat 30 ml of oil over medium heat.
- Mix in the garlic and ginger. 1 minute of sautéing
- Combine the broth, lemongrass, chilli paste, shiitake mushrooms, and cherry tomatoes in a mixing bowl.
- Bring everything to a low heat and cook for 12-15 minutes, or until the mushrooms are soft.
- While the soup cooks, chop the tofu into 12 inch pieces.
- Heat the remaining 15 ml of oil in a medium skillet over medium-high heat.
- Arrange the tofu cubes in a single layer on a baking sheet.
- Cook for about 5 minutes, or until the bottoms are lightly browned, then flip and cook for another 5 minutes.
- Toss in the tofu.
- Stir in the tofu, cilantro, and lime juice after adding it to the broth mixture.
- To taste, season with soy sauce.
- Remove and discard the lemongrass pieces.
- Pour into bowls and serve.

Nutrient value: Per serving
- Calories: 136 kcal
- Carbohydrates: 7 g
- Protein: 10 g
- Fat: 7 g

---

3. SOUP WITH SPICY SRIRACHA LIME CHICKEN ZOODLE

Prep Time: 2 minutes
Cook Time: 13 minutes
Servings: 2 people

Ingredients:
- 250 g chicken breast (approx. 1 large)
- 1 L broth (chicken or vegetable)
- 1 g garlic powder
- 1 g cumin
- 1 medium zucchini squash
- 3 ml fresh lime juice
- 15 g fresh chopped cilantro
- 5 g Sriracha, plus more to taste
- 2 lime slices/wedges

Directions:
- Slice the chicken and place it in a pot over medium-high heat.
- Bring broth, garlic powder [or raw garlic!] and cumin to a boil.
- Once the water is boiling, decrease the heat to low and simmer for 10 minutes, or until the chicken is well cooked.
- While the chicken is cooking, use a spiralizer to make excellent zucchini noodles.
- When the chicken is done, add the zucchini noodles and lime juice to the soup and continue to cook for 3 minutes, or until the desired tenderness is obtained. Cook the noodles for a few minutes longer if you want softer noodles.
- Divide the soup between two big bowls and top with fresh cilantro and a generous drizzle of Sriracha chilli sauce.
- You can add a little or a lot! I use a lot of garlic in mine.
- Serve with lime wedges

Nutrient value: Per serving
- Calories: 172 kcal
- Carbohydrates: 3 g
- Protein: 9 g
- Fat: 27 g

---

4. SOUP WITH HAM AND CABBAGE IN AN INSTANT POT

Prep Time: 15 minutes
Cook Time: 15 minutes
 Servings: 8 people

Ingredients:
- 1 cabbage head, chopped

- 250 g finely chopped onion
- 1 finely chopped red bell pepper
- 2 small carrots, sliced in small rounds or minced
- 450 g diced lean ham
- 2 bay leaves
- 3 g Spike Seasoning
- 10 g granulated garlic
- 13 g dried parsley
- 3 g Beau Monde Seasoning or coarse crushed black pepper to taste
- two packets Goya Ham Flavor Concentrate or a different ham flavour base

Directions:
- Chop the cabbage, onion, red bell pepper, ham, and carrots into small pieces (if using).
- In the bottom of the Instant Pot, combine the cabbage, onion, and red bell pepper. Sprinkle the Spike Seasoning, granulated garlic, dry parsley, Beau Monde Seasoning, and black pepper over the diced ham, carrots, and bay leaves.
- Pour the liquid over the ingredients in the Instant Pot after mixing the Goya Ham Flavor Concentrate or other ham flavour base into the chicken stock.
- Lock the cover and cook for 15 minutes on MANUAL, HIGH PRESSURE.
- Allow for NATURAL RELEASE for 10-15 minutes before releasing manually.
- Serve immediately, with freshly grated Parmesan on the side if desired.

Nutrient value: Per serving
- Calories: 241 kcal
- Carbohydrates: 7 g
- Protein: 26 g
- Fat: 8 g

---

5. Soup With Chipotle Shrimp Tacos

Prep Time: 15 minutes
Cook Time: 25 minutes
Servings: 4 people

Ingredients:
- 450 g shrimp, thawed with tails removed
- Tomatoes, crushed (750 g)
- 120 g chopped white onion
- 20 g minced garlic
- 1 serrano or jalapeo chilli pepper, chopped
- 1 L low sodium chicken broth
- 250 ml of water
- 3 g onion powder
- 3 g oregano
- 10 g chipotle powder
- 3 g cumin
- 2 g ground coriander

Directions:
- In a large 7 L saucepan, saute the onion, garlic, and diced chilli pepper over medium heat.
- Cook for 2-3 minutes, stirring periodically, until softened.
- Stir in the spices to the saucepan.
- Then combine the diced tomatoes, broth, and water in a mixing bowl.
- Bring the pot to a boil, then reduce to a low simmer.
- Cover the pot with the shrimp.
- Cook for another 10-15 minutes on a low heat until the shrimp are opaque.
- When the shrimp is done, plate them.

Nutrient value:
Per serving
- Calories: 211 kcal
- Carbohydrates: 20g
- Protein: 28 g
- Fat: 2 g

---

6. Soup With Smoked Turkey Sausage

Prep Time: 15 minutes
Cook Time: 45 minutes
Servings: 6 people

Ingredients:

- 30 ml extra-virgin olive oil
- 1 medium diced onion
- 1 medium peeled and diced sweet potato, cut into 1/2 inch cubes
- 450 g smoked turkey sausage, cut into 3/4-inch rounds
- 1 L chicken stock containers
- 2 g dried oregano
- 1 g dried rosemary
- 3 g minced garlic
- 120 g fresh spinach
- Season with salt and pepper to taste.

Directions:
- Warm the olive oil in the bottom of a large stock-pot over medium heat.
- Cook until the onion is transparent but not browned, about 2 minutes.
- Cook for a few minutes more after adding the turkey sausage rounds.
- Pour in the chicken stock and whisk to include the onions and sausage.
- Stir in the sweet potato, oregano, rosemary, and garlic until well combined.
- Bring the soup to a low boil and continue to cook for about 15 minutes.
- Reduce the heat to low and continue to cook the soup for another 15-20 minutes.
- Like any soup, the longer it simmers, the more condensed and tasty it becomes.
- Add the fresh spinach and mix well.
- Season with salt and pepper and serve

Nutrient value: Per serving
- Calories: 130 kcal
- Carbohydrates: 2 g
- Protein: 4 g
- Fat: 5 g

7. CREOLE CORN SOUP

Prep Time: 15 minutes
Cook Time: 1 hour 10 minutes

Servings: 6 people

Ingredients:
- 120 ml vegetable oil
- 90 g all-purpose flour
- 2 medium sliced onions
- 2 minced garlic cloves
- 700 g stewed tomatoes, undrained and mashed
- 250 g tomatoes with green chile peppers
- 400 g cream-style corn
- 400 g whole kernel corn
- 1 L low-sodium chicken broth (or unsalted chicken broth)
- 900 g shrimp, to taste, preferably
- Fresh Kosher salt
- To taste, freshly ground black pepper

Directions:
- Warm the vegetable oil in a large saucepan or stockpot over medium-low heat.
- Cook, stirring constantly, until the roux reaches a light yellow colour.
- Make sure it doesn't get too dark.
- Cook until the onions and garlic are softened, about 5 minutes.
- Cook for 45 minutes over low heat with the stewed tomatoes, tomatoes with chiles, cream-style corn, whole kernel corn, and broth.
- In the meantime, peel the shrimp. Remove the dark vein from the back of a shrimp with the point of a small, sharp knife.
- Rep with the rest of the prawns.
- Continue to cook for about 10 minutes after adding the shrimp to the soup mixture.
- Season with kosher salt and freshly ground black pepper to taste.

Nutrient value: Per serving
- Calories: 686 kcal
- Carbohydrates: 6 g
- Protein: 48 g
- Fat: 25 g

Prep Time: 15 minutes
Cook Time: 5 minutes
Servings: 6 people

Ingredients:

- Pumpkin (225 g)
- 2 onions, red
- 1 yellow bell pepper, chopped
- 1/4 broccoli head (discard the stem)
- 2 celery spears
- 10 little cherry tomatoes
- 1 L of hot water
- 60 ml soy sauce or tamari
- 3 g ginger powder
- 10 g garlic powder
- 10 g onion powder
- 10 g Provence herbs
- 20 g nutritional yeast
- To taste, lemon juice

Directions:

- Spiralize the pumpkin or finely cut it with a knife.
- A peeler can also be used.
- Place the remaining vegetables in a large pot with the pumpkin. Combine the water, soy sauce, spices (ginger, garlic, and onion powder), and herbs in a mixing bowl.
- Cook for 5 to 10 minutes over medium-high heat.
- When the soup is finished, add the nutritional yeast and lemon juice right before serving, stir, and serve!

Nutrient value: Per serving

- Calories: 130 kcal
- Carbohydrates: 0 g
- Protein: 3 g
- Fat: 5 g

Prep Time: 10 minutes
Cook Time: 20 minutes

Servings: 5 people

Ingredients:

- Asparagus 450 g asparagus, chopped
- 1 chopped fennel bulb
- 120 g fresh basil
- 750 ml vegetable broth
- 1 chopped yellow onion
- 3 minced garlic cloves
- 30 ml olive oil
- seasoned with salt & pepper
- Optional garnish: pepita olive oil
- If you're vegan, leave out the yoghurt

Directions:

- Heat the olive oil in a big pot over medium-high heat.
- Sauté the chopped onion and fennel for 5 minutes, or until softened.
- Cook for a minute, or until the garlic is aromatic, before adding the minced garlic.
- Add the broth, cover, and cook for 10 minutes on low heat.
- Cook for 2 minutes over low heat after adding the chopped asparagus.
- Remove from the heat and, once somewhat cooled, combine with the basil until the soup is creamy and smooth.
- Return to the stove over low heat and season with salt and pepper.
- Serve the soup while it is still hot, garnished if desired.

Nutrient value: Per serving

- Calories: 113 kcal
- Carbohydrates: 9 g
- Protein: 5 g
- Fat: 6 g

Prep Time: 10 minutes
Cook Time: 18 minutes
Servings: 4 people

Ingredients:
- 2 medium peeled and spiralized potatoes
- 1 large or 2 small spiralized zucchini
- 1 carrot, peeled and spiralized
- 1 celery root, peeled and spiralized the size of a medium potato
- 1 finely chopped onion
- 30 ml olive oil
- 850-900 ml hot vegetable stock
- Garnish with fresh dill and/or parsley
- season with pepper to taste

Directions:
- In a medium-sized pot, heat 30 ml of oil and gently sauté the onions for 3 minutes, or until softened (but not browned), turning often.
- Continue cooking for 4 minutes over a low/medium heat, stirring frequently, with the spiralized carrot, celeriac, and potato.
- Spiralize the zucchini, add the stock, and season with pepper to taste.
- Cover and bring to a boil, then reduce to a low heat and continue to cook for 3 minutes, stirring regularly.
- Remove from the fire, stir in the chopped herbs, season to taste, and serve.

Nutrient value: Per serving
- Calories: 98nkcal
- Carbohydrates: 8 g
- Protein: 1 g
- Fat: 7 g

---

11. Soup With Roast Cauliflower And Kale

Prep Time: 20 minutes
Cook Time: 40 minutes
Servings: 6 people

Ingredients:
- 1 large cauliflower head, trimmed and divided into florets
- 4 big peeled garlic cloves
- Extra virgin olive oil
- salt kosher
- black pepper, freshly ground
- 1 large bunch kale, rough stems removed, cut into 1 inch pieces and divided
- 1.5 L vegetable or chicken stock
- 1 medium onion, diced
- Pine nuts, toasted
- Olive oil (extra virgin)

Directions:
- Preheat the oven to 218°C.
- Combine the cauliflower and garlic in a bowl with a few ml olive oil.
- Season with salt and pepper to taste.
- Place on a baking sheet in a single layer.
- Cook for about 20 minutes, or until the cauliflower is soft and golden.
- Stir seldom. Check to see whether the garlic is browning too soon. If this is the case, remove from the pan.
- Remove from the oven and reduce the temperature to 165°C.
- Toss half of the kale with about a tablespoon of olive oil in a mixing bowl.
- Season with salt and pepper to taste. Put them on a baking pan.
- Roast for about 25 minutes, stirring halfway through, until the kale is crispy.
- In a heavy pot or Dutch oven, heat about 30 ml olive oil over medium heat while the kale is baking.
- Cook, turning occasionally, until the onion is transparent and tender, about 5 minutes.
- Add the cauliflower, garlic, and stock to the pot. Bring the water to a boil. Reduce the heat to medium-low, cover, and leave to cook for 10 minutes.
- Stir in the rest of the kale. Return the heat to medium and cook for 5 minutes. In a blender, purée the soup in batches until smooth.
- Return to the pot.
- Ladle into heated bowls to serve. Top with crispy kale, pine nuts, and a drizzle of extra virgin olive oil.

Nutrient value: Per serving
- Calories: 330 kcal
- Carbohydrates: 10 g
- Protein: 29 g
- Fat: 15 g

---

12. IMMUNE-BOOSTING SOUP

Prep Time: 5 minutes
Cook Time: 1 hour 30 minutes
Servings: 8 people

Ingredients:
- 15 ml coconut oil
- 1 large yellow onion, minced
- 6 garlic cloves,
- 2 celery stalks, sliced
- 450 g of shiitake mushrooms
- 5 g sea salt
- 1 g black pepper
- 3 g turmeric
- 3 L water
- 4 baby bok choy heads, bottoms removed
- Optional: 1/2 head chopped kale
- 10 g ginger, freshly grated

Directions:
- Remove and discard the very bottom of the mushroom stem. Separate the stems from the tops and, if necessary, cut the tops and remaining stem into large pieces. You will only discard the very bottom of the stems, not the entire stems, because they offer numerous nutritional benefits!
- In a large pot over medium heat, melt the coconut oil.
- Cook for 5 minutes, or until the onions are transparent.
- Cook for 1 minute more after adding the garlic.
- Sauté the celery and mushrooms for about 10 minutes, or until the mushrooms have wilted.
- Bring the spices (including the ginger, if using) and water to a boil.
- Then, cover and leave to boil for 1 hour or as long as you like (the longer you leave, the better!)
- Wilt the bok choy and kale in the last 10 minutes of cooking.
- Serve warm or store in the refrigerator for up to 1 week.

Nutrient value: Per serving
- Calories: 230 kcal
- Carbohydrates: 8 g
- Protein: 32 g
- Fat: 25 g

---

13. CARROT GINGER SOUP

Prep Time: 10 minutes
Cook Time: 1 hour 40 minutes
Servings: 5 people

Ingredients:
- 15 ml avocado oil
- 450 g carrots, chopped
- 450 g onion (roughly chopped)
- 10 g ginger (grated)
- 7 ml lemon zest
- 30 g golden raisins (or any other variety)
- 2 g sea salt (or any other kind)
- 100 ml homemade veggie broth
- 30 g almonds

Directions:
- Preheat the oven to 202 C. Place the carrots and onion in a single layer in a baking dish
- To the vegetables, add 75 ml vegetable broth and 1 g salt.
- Mix by hand to coat the vegetables evenly.
- Cook for 45-60 minutes in a preheated oven.
- 5 ml oil, heated in a heavy-bottom soup pot over medium heat
- Stir in the ginger and simmer for 10 seconds in the oil.
- Combine oven-roasted carrots and onions, 2 g salt, 1 L vegetable broth, lemon zest, and golden raisins in a mixing bowl. Bring the soup to a gentle simmer over medium heat (approximately 10-12 minutes) and cook

for a further 10 minutes.
- Remove the soup from the oven.
- Remove the soup from the heat and set it aside to cool completely.
- In a blender, puree the soup. Check to see if there are any pesky veggie bits remaining in the soup.
- Toast almonds lightly in a toaster or on the stove-top in a heavy-bottom skillet.
- Serve with a bean salad!

Nutrient value: Per serving
- Calories: 110 kcal
- Carbohydrates: 10 g
- Protein: 2 g
- Fat: 5 g

---

14. PEPPER TOMATO SOUP

Prep Time: 10 minutes
Cook Time: 30 minutes
Servings: 4 people

Ingredients:
- 4 bell peppers, red
- three huge tomatoes
- 1 medium onion
- 5 cloves garlic
- 175 g tomato paste
- 15 ml balsamic vinegar
- 3 g dried basil
- 350 ml liquid (stock or water)
- 45 ml olive oil,
- Salt, and pepper to taste

GARNISH
- the oil of olives
- fresh basil, black pepper, hemp seeds

Directions:
- Set your oven's top broiler to broil.
- Half the red bell peppers, tomatoes, and onion.
- Remove the seeds and stems from the bell peppers, as well as the stems and outer peel from the tomatoes and onion.
- Place everything on a baking sheet, sprinkle with olive oil, and season with salt and pepper.
- Rub the oil and seasoning into both sides of the vegetables with your fingertips.
- Roast the vegetables for 25-30 minutes, or until the top is blackened and charred.
- Transfer the bell pepper to a glass bowl with tongs and cover with plastic wrap for about 20 minutes to steam.
- When the other vegetables are cold enough to handle, remove their skins and place them in a Vitamix or other high-powered blender.
- You should also be able to easily squeeze the garlic cloves from their peel.
- In a blender, combine the tomato paste, balsamic vinegar, dried basil, and water (or stock). Blend on high until everything is smooth.
- The soup will be heated at this point.
- Blend for another 4-5 minutes if you want it hotter.
- The friction of the blades in the Vitamix will heat it up.
- Garnish with optional garnish before serving.

Nutrient value: Per serving
- Calories: 223 kcal
- Carbohydrates: 4 g
- Protein: 24 g
- Fat: 11 g

---

15. SOUP WITH SPINACH AND EGG DROPS

Prep Time: 15 minutes
Cook Time: 45 minutes
Servings: 4 people

Ingredients:
- 30 ml olive oil
- 450 g fresh baby spinach
- 1 garlic clove, pressed
- 1 carrot, peeled and cut into small cubes or shredded

- 45 g chopped green onion
- 10 g ground black pepper
- 1 cube chicken bullion — or to taste,
- 10 g Vegetta salt
- 30 g tomato sauce
- 1 L water
- 2 beaten eggs + 30 ml water
- 30 ml lemon juice

Directions:

- Cook spinach in olive oil for 5 minutes in a large pot over medium heat.
- Cook for 3 minutes more after adding the garlic and carrot.
- Stir in the black pepper, tomato sauce, water, and chicken bullion. Cook the soup for 30 minutes on medium heat.
- Stir in the egg and water mixture slowly until the eggs are fully cooked.
- Pour in the lemon juice. Season with salt to taste. Garnish with green onion slices.

Nutrient value: Per serving

- Calories: 111 kcal
- Carbohydrates: 4 g
- Protein: 3 g
- Fat: 9 g

CHAPTER 17

RECIPES MEAT

1. Meatballs With Keto Sauce

Prep Time: 30 minutes
Cook Time: 15 minutes
Servings: 4 people

Ingredients:
- 120 g Parmesan cheese, grated
- 120 g of shredded mozzarella cheese
- 1 big, lightly beaten egg
- 30 g heavy whipping cream
- 1 minced garlic clove
- 450 g ground beef, lean (90 percent lean)

Sauce
- 220 g basil, garlic, and oregano tomato sauce
- 30 g pesto (prepared)
- 1 kg heavy whipping cream

Directions:
- Preheat the oven to 176⁰C.
- Combine the first five ingredients in a large mixing bowl.
- Mix in the beef lightly but thoroughly.
- Form into 1-1/2-inch balls.
- Place the meatballs in a 15x10x1-inch baking pan on a greased rack.
- Bake for 15-20 minutes, or until thoroughly done.
- Meanwhile, combine the sauce ingredients in a small saucepan and boil through.
- Serve with meatballs if desired.

Nutrient value: Per four meat balls
- Calories: 404 kcal
- Carbohydrates: 7 g
- Protein: 31 g
- Fat: 27 g

2. Smothered Chicken

Prep Time: 10 minutes
Cook Time: 20 minutes
Servings: 4 people

Ingredients:
- 10 ml olive oil
- 200 g fresh mushrooms, sliced
- 3 sliced green onions
- 700 g baby spinach, fresh
- 30 g pecans, chopped
- 4 chicken breast halves, boneless and skinless (150 g each)
- 3 g rotisserie chicken seasoning
- 2 halved slices reduced-fat provolone cheese

Directions:
- Preheat the grill or the broiler. Heat oil in a large skillet over medium-high heat; sauté mushrooms and green onions until tender.
- Stir in the spinach and pecans until wilted.
- Remove from the heat and keep warm.
- Season the chicken to taste.
- Grill, covered, over medium heat on an oiled grill

rack or broil 4 in. from the fire on a greased broiler pan until a thermometer reads 73°C, 4-5 minutes each side.
- Top with cheese and grill or broil until melted.
- To serve, spoon the mushroom mixture over top.

Nutrient value: Per serving
- Calories: 203 kcal
- Carbohydrates: 3 g
- Protein: 27 g
- Fat: 9 g

3. RUBBED CHICKEN THIGHS

Prep Time: 5 minutes
Cook Time: 15 minutes
Servings: 6 people

Ingredients:
- 3 g sea salt
- 3 g garlic powder
- 3 g onions powder
- 3 g dried oregano
- 3 g turmeric powder
- 1 g paprika
- 1 g chilli powder
- 1 g pepper
- 6 boneless skinless chicken thighs (about 600 g)

Directions:
- Combine the first 8 ingredients in a small mixing dish.
- Sprinkle evenly over both sides of the chicken.
- Grill chicken, covered, over medium heat or broil 4 in. from heat until a thermometer reads 75°C, 6-8 minutes per side, on a lightly greased grill rack.

Nutrient value: Per piece
- Calories: 169 kcal
- Carbohydrates: 1 g
- Protein: 21 g
- Fat: 8 g

4. THIGHS OF CHICKEN WITH SHALLOTS AND SPINACH

Prep Time: 10 minutes
Cook Time: 20 minutes
Servings: 6 people

Ingredients:
- 6 boneless skinless chicken thighs (about 600 g)
- 2 g of seasoned salt
- 2 g black pepper
- 3 ml olive oil
- 4 finely sliced shallots
- 100 ml white wine or chicken broth (low sodium)
- a single packet (250 g) trimmed fresh spinach
- 1 g salt
- 75 g low-fat sour cream

Directions:
- Season the chicken with salt and pepper.
- Heat the oil in a large nonstick skillet over medium heat.
- Cook until the chicken reaches a temperature of 70°C, about 6 minutes per side.
- Remove from pan and set aside to keep heated.
- Cook and stir shallots in the same pan until tender.
- Bring the wine to a boil.
- Cook until the wine has been reduced by half.
- Cook, stirring constantly, until the spinach is wilted.
- Stir in the sour cream and serve with the chicken.
- Cool the chicken and spinach combination before adding the sour cream. Freeze in ice cube trays. To use, defrost slightly in the refrigerator overnight. In a covered skillet, heat slowly, stirring periodically, until a thermometer inserted into the chicken reads 170°. Sour cream should be added last.

Nutrient value: Per piece
- Calories: 223 kcal
- Carbohydrates: 7 g
- Protein: 23 g
- Fat: 10 g

Prep Time: 10 minutes
Cook Time: 7 hour
Servings: 15 people

Ingredients:
- 2 boneless beef chuck roasts (each 1 kg)
- 1 package ranch salad dressing mix
- 1 enveloppe salad dressing mix (Italian)
- 1 package brown gravy mix
- 120 ml water
- Optional: chopped fresh parsley

Directions:
- In a 5 L slow cooker, place the chuck roasts.
- Combine the salad dressings and gravy mix in a small dish; stir in the water. Pour over the meat.
- Cook on low for 7-8 hours, or until the vegetables are soft.
- Sprinkle with parsley and thicken cooking liquids for gravy if desired.

Nutrient value: Per serving
- Calories: 142 kcal
- Carbohydrates: 3 g
- Protein: 15 g
- Fat: 7 g

Prep Time: 10 minutes
Cook Time: 10 minutes
Servings: 4 people

Ingredients:
- a single packet (550 g) Tenderloins of turkey breast
- 3 g chicken seasoning
- 1 g of seasoned salt
- 1 g pepper, split
- 30 ml canola oil
- 10 g melted butter
- 100 g all-purpose flour
- 450 ml chicken stock

Directions:
- Tenderloins should be cut into 1-inch slices cross-wise; flatten pieces with a meat mallet to 1/2-inch thickness.
- Combine poultry seasoning, seasoned salt, and 1 g pepper in a small bowl; sprinkle over turkey.
- Heat the oil in a large skillet over medium-high heat.
- Cook the turkey in batches until it is no longer pink, about 2-3 minutes per side. Remove from pan and set aside to keep heated.
- Melt butter in the same pan over medium heat; whisk in flour until smooth. Stir in the broth gradually.
- Bring to a boil; cook and stir for 2 minutes, or until thickened.
- Finish with the remaining pepper.
- Serve with roasted turkey.

Nutrient value: Per serving
- Calories: 292 kcal
- Carbohydrates: 7 g
- Protein: 31 g
- Fat: 15 g

Prep Time: 15 minutes
Cook Time: 4 hours
Servings: 6 people

Ingredients:
- 5 g salt
- 1 g pepper
- 1 g paprika
- 15 g lemon-pepper seasoning
- 6 bone-in, skin-removed chicken breast halves (200 g each)
- 250 g undiluted condensed cream of mushroom soup
- 1 Kg sour cream
- 120 ml chicken broth or dry white wine

- 220 g fresh sliced mushrooms
- 250 ml of water
- 30 ml cornstarch
- Optional additional paprika

Directions:
- Combine the first four ingredients in a small bowl; rub over the chicken.
- Fill a 3-quart slow cooker halfway with water.
- Combine the soup, sour cream, and wine in a large mixing bowl; whisk in the mushrooms. Drizzle over the chicken.
- Cook on low for 4 hours, or until the meat is soft.
- In a separate bowl, whisk together the water and cornstarch until smooth; add into the chicken mixture.
- Return to a boil, stirring continually, until the sauce thickens.
- Sprinkle with more paprika if desired.

Nutrient value: Per Piece
- Calories: 317 kcal
- Carbohydrates: 6 g
- Protein: 26 g
- Fat: 13 g

---

8. CHICKEN GARLIC WHITE WINE

Prep Time: 10 minutes
Cook Time: 20 minutes
Servings: 4 people

Ingredients:
- 4 chicken breast halves, boneless and skinless (200 g each)
- 1 g pepper
- 2 g salt
- 5 ml olive oil
- 450 g baby portobello mushrooms, sliced
- 1 medium sliced onion
- 2 minced garlic cloves
- 120 ml dry white wine or chicken broth (low sodium)

Directions:
- Pound chicken breasts to 1/2-inch thickness with a meat mallet; season with salt and pepper.
- Heat the oil in a large skillet over medium heat; cook the chicken until it is no longer pink, 5-6 minutes per side.
- Remove from pan and set aside to keep heated.
- Cook and stir mushrooms and onion in pan over medium-high heat until soft and faintly browned, 2-3 minutes.
- Cook and stir for 30 seconds after adding the garlic.
- Bring wine to a boil, stirring to release browned pieces from the pan.
- Cook until the liquid is somewhat reduced, about 1-2 minutes; serve with the chicken.

Nutrient value: Per serving
- Calories: 243 kcal
- Carbohydrates: 5 g
- Protein: 36 g
- Fat: 7 g

---

9. PROVOLONE CHICKEN CHEESE

Prep Time: 5 minutes
Cook Time: 20 minutes
Servings: 4 people

Ingredients:
- 4 chicken breast halves, boneless and skinless (150 g each)
- 1 g pepper
- Cooking spray scented with butter
- 8 basil leaves, fresh
- 4 slices prosciutto or deli ham, thinly sliced
- 4 provolone cheese slices

Directions:
- Season the chicken with pepper.
- Cook the chicken in a large skillet sprayed with cooking spray over medium heat until a thermometer

reads 73°C, about 4-5 minutes each side.
- Transfer to a baking sheet that hasn't been oiled; top with the basil, prosciutto, and cheese.
- Broil 6-8 inches from the flame until the cheese melts, about 1-2 minutes.

Nutrient value: Per serving
- Calories: 236 kcal
- Carbohydrates: 1 g
- Protein: 33 g
- Fat: 11 g

---

10. Roasted Beef With Gravy

Prep Time: 15 minutes
Cook Time: 8 hours
Servings: 10 people

Ingredients:
- 1 boneless chuck roast beef (1.5 Kg)
- 2 tins (280 g) undiluted condensed cream of mushroom soup
- 100 ml sherry or beef broth
- 1 onion soup mix envelope

Directions:
- Cut the roast in half and set it in a 3 L slow cooker.
- Combine the other ingredients in a large mixing bowl; pour over the roast.
- Cook on low for 8-10 hours, or until the meat is soft.
- Optional freezing: Place sliced pot roast in freezer containers and top with cooking liquids. Allow to cool and freeze. To use, defrost slightly in the refrigerator overnight. In a covered pot, heat through, slowly stirring and adding a little water as needed.

Nutrient value: Per serving
- Calories: 267 kcal
- Carbohydrates: 4 g
- Protein: 28 g
- Fat: 14 g

11. Steak with Rolled Flanks

Prep Time: 45 minutes
Cook Time: 1 hour
Servings: 6 people

Ingredients:
- 60 ml soy sauce
- 900 g beef flank steak
- 120 ml extra virgin olive oil
- 7 g spice for steak
- 250 g provolone cheese, thinly sliced
- 4 thick-cut bacon pieces
- 120 g FRESH SPROUTING
- 120 g crimini mushrooms, sliced
- 450 g red bell pepper, seeded and sliced into strips

Directions:
- On a cutting board, place the flank steak with the short end closest to you. Cut through the flesh horizontally from one of the long sides to within 1/2 inch of the opposite edge.
- In a gallon-sized resealable plastic bag, combine the soy sauce, olive oil, and steak seasoning.
- Refrigerate the flank steak for 4 hours to overnight.
- Preheat the oven to 176°C.
- Grease a glass baking dish with cooking spray.
- Lay the flank steak flat in front of you, grain going from left to right.
- Provolone should be layered across the steak, leaving a 1-inch border.
- Place the bacon, spinach, red pepper, and mushrooms in stripes across the cheese-covered steak in the same direction.
- Roll the flank steak up and away from you so that each of the filler components can be seen when the roll is cut into a pinwheel form.
- Roll tightly, but avoid squeezing the fillings out the ends.
- Tie kitchen twine every 2 inches after the roll is complete.
- Bake for one hour, or until the internal temperature reaches 65°C, in a preheated oven. Remove from

the oven and set aside to cool for 5–10 minutes before slicing into 1 inch slices.
• Before serving, make sure the string is removed.

Nutrition fact: Per serving
• Calories: 413 kcal
• Carbohydrates: 5 g
• Protein: 31 g
• Fats: 36 g

---

11. Foil-Wrapped Pot Roast

Prep Time: 10 minutes
Cook Time: 4 hour
Servings: 8 people

Ingredients:
• 300 g condensed cream of mushroom soup
• 1.5 kg bottom round
• 1 packet onion soup mix (dry)
• 20 ml of water

Directions:
• Preheat the oven to 150⁰C.
• In the bottom of a 9x13 inch roasting pan, place a 30 inch long sheet of foil. In the pan, place the roast on the foil.
• Combine the mushroom soup and onion soup mix in a separate small bowl. Combine all of the ingredients in a large mixing bowl and pour over the roast. Using the water, spritz the area. Fold the foil in half and secure the edges.
• Preheat oven to 150⁰C and bake for 4 hours.

Nutrition fact: Per serving
• Calories: 389 kcal
• Carbohydrates: 3 g
• Protein: 35 g
• Fats: 25 g

---

12. Beef Tenderloin With Blue Cheese

Prep Time: 30 minutes
Cook Time: 1 hour
Servings: 8 people

Ingredients:
• 120 g teriyaki sauce
• 1.5 kg entire beef tenderloin
• 450 ml red wine
• 120 g blue cheese, crumbled
• 2 garlic cloves, diced
• 100 g of mayonnaise
• 100 g of sour cream
• 5 g Worcestershire sauce

Directions:
• In a shallow dish, place the beef. Combine the teriyaki sauce, red wine, and garlic in a mixing bowl; pour over the beef. Allow beef to marinade for 30 minutes in the refrigerator.
• Preheat the oven to 230⁰C.
• Place tenderloin on broiler pan and cook for 15 minutes in a preheated oven. Reduce the heat to 190⁰C and continue to cook for another 30 to 40 minutes, or until desired doneness is reached. Allow 10 minutes to set before slicing.
• Combine blue cheese, mayonnaise, sour cream, and Worcestershire sauce in a skillet over low heat. Serve over sliced tenderloin after stirring until smooth.

Nutrition fact: Per serving
• Calories: 669 kcal
• Carbohydrates: 5 g
• Protein: 35 g
• Fats: 54 g

---

13. Brisket With Barbecue Sauce

Prep Time: 10 minutes
Cook Time: 6 hour
Servings: 10 people

Ingredients:

- 2 kg brisket of lean beef
- 10 ml liquid smoke flavour
- 10 g salt for onions
- 10 g salt (garlic)
- 15 g brown sugar
- ketchup, 250 g
- 45 g unsalted butter
- 60 ml of water
- 3 g celery salt
- 10 g liquid smokiness
- 20 g WORCESTERSHIRE SEASONING
- 7 g powdered mustard
- season with salt and pepper to taste

Directions:

- Smoke the brisket with liquid smoke. Season with onion and garlic salt. Wrap the brisket in foil and place it in the refrigerator overnight.
- Preheat the oven to 150⁰C.
- In a large roasting pan, place the beef. Bake for 5 to 6 hours, covered. Remove from the oven, allow to cool before slicing. Return the slices to the pan.
- Combine brown sugar, ketchup, butter, water, celery salt, liquid smoke, Worcestershire sauce, mustard, salt, and pepper in a medium pot. Cook, stirring constantly, until the water boils.
- Pour the sauce on top of the meat slices in the pan. Bake for another hour, covered.

Nutrition fact: Per serving

- Calories: 560 kcal
- Carbohydrates: 9 g
- Protein: 34 g
- Fats: 42 g

14. COOKER BARBEQUE

Prep Time: 10 minutes
Cook Time: 9 hour
Servings: 8 people

Ingredients:

- Boneless chuck roast, 1.5 kg
- 3 g powdered garlic
- 3 g powdered onion
- season with salt and pepper to taste
- 1 bottle barbeque sauce, 450 ml

Directions:

- In a slow cooker, place the roast.
- Season with salt and pepper and a pinch of garlic and onion powder.
- Barbeque sauce should be poured over the meat.
- Cook for 6 to 8 hours on low.
- Remove the meat from the slow cooker, shred it, and put it back in.
- Cook for a another hour. Serve immediately.

Nutrition fact: Per serving

- Calories: 344 kcal
- Carbohydrates: 23 g
- Protein: 17 g
- Fats: 36 g

15. ROAST SIRLOIN WITH GRAVY

Prep Time: 20 minutes
Cook Time: 3 ½ hours
Servings: 8 people

Ingredients:

- 1 roast beef sirloin tip (1.5 kg)
- 2 minced garlic cloves
- 20 g coarsely ground pepper
- 75 ml low-sodium soy sauce
- 45 ml balsamic vinaigrette
- 3 ml Worcestershire sauce
- 20 g mustard powder
- 20 g cornstarch
- 75 ml of cold water

Directions:

- Place the roast in a 3 L slow cooker and season with garlic and pepper.
- Pour over the roast the mixture of soy sauce, vine-

gar, Worcestershire sauce, and mustard.
- Cook, covered, on low heat for 3 1/2 to 4 hours, or until vegetables are soft.
- Keep the roast heated.
- Cooking liquids should be strained into a small saucepan; fat should be skimmed off.
- Stir cornstarch and water together until smooth; add to cooking liquids.
- Bring to a boil; cook and stir for 1-2 minutes, or until thickened.
- Serve the roast in pieces with gravy.

Nutrient value: Per serving
- Calories: 241 kcal
- Carbohydrates: 5 g
- Protein: 35 g
- Fat: 8 g

---

16. BACON-WRAPS

Prep Time: 10 minutes
Cook Time: 20 minutes
Servings: 2 people

Ingredients:
- 10 stalks fresh asparagus, trimmed Cooking spray
- 1 g black pepper
- 5 bacon pieces, cut in half lengthwise

Directions:
- Arrange the asparagus on a sheet of waxed paper and spray with cooking spray. Season with pepper and toss to coat.
- Wrap a strip of bacon around each spear and attach with toothpicks.
- Grill, uncovered, over medium heat for 4-6 minutes per side until bacon is crisp.
- Throw away the toothpicks.

Nutrient value: 4 pieces
- Calories: 120 kcal
- Carbohydrates: 4 g
- Protein: 9 g
- Fat: 8 g

17. SAVORY RUBBED ROAST CHICKEN

Prep Time: 20 minutes
Cook Time: 2 hours
Servings: 12 people

Ingredients:
- 2 paprika teaspoons
- 3 g salt,
- 3 g onion powder
- 3 g ground white pepper
- 3 g cayenne pepper
- 3 g dried thyme
- 1 g garlic powder
- 2 g black pepper
- 1 chicken, roasted (3 kg)
- 1 large onion, peeled and sliced into wedges

Directions:
- Preheat the oven to 176⁰C.
- Combine the first eight ingredients in a small mixing dish.
- Pat the chicken dry and arrange it breast side up on a rack in a roasting pan.
- Rub the seasoning mixture all over the chicken, both inside and out.
- Place the onion inside the hollow.
- Tuck the wings under the chicken and knot the drumsticks together.
- Roast for 2 to 2-1/2 hours, or until a thermometer inserted into the thickest portion of the thigh registers 170°C-175°C. (If the chicken browns too soon, cover loosely with foil.) Remove the chicken from the oven and tent with foil.
- Allow to stand for 15 minutes before carving.

Nutrient value: Per serving
- Calories: 272 kcal
- Carbohydrates: 2 g
- Protein: 29g
- Fat: 16 g

Prep Time: 5 minutes
Cook Time: 30 minutes
Servings: 6 people

Ingredients:
*   6 boneless, skinless chicken breast half-hundredths (120 g each)
*   1 g paprika
*   15 g butter
*   250 g fresh mushrooms, sliced
*   120 g sherry or chicken broth
*   3 sliced green onions
*   1 minced garlic clove
*   2 g of salt
*   1 g black pepper
*   60 g part-skim mozzarella cheese, shredded

Directions:
*   Place the chicken in a 13x9-inch baking dish that has been sprayed with cooking spray. Garnish with paprika. Bake for 15 minutes, uncovered, at 176°C.
*   Meanwhile, sauté mushrooms in butter in a large nonstick skillet for 5 minutes.
*   Combine the sherry or broth, green onions, garlic, salt, and pepper in a mixing bowl.
*   Bring the water to a boil. Drizzle over the chicken.
*   Bake for 10-15 minutes more, or until a thermometer reads 76°C.
*   Serve with cheese on top. Bake for 3-5 minutes, or until the cheese melts.

Nutrient value: Per serving
*   Calories: 215 kcal
*   Carbohydrates: 6 g
*   Protein: 28 g
*   Fat: 8 g

Prep Time: 20 minutes
Cook Time: 40 minutes

Servings: 12 people

Ingredients:
*   5 ml olive oil
*   3 kg bone-in short ribs of beef
*   30 g melted butter
*   1 medium leek, coarsely chopped (just the white portion)
*   1 minced garlic clove
*   250 ml chicken broth
*   a single can (170 g) tomato puree
*   20 g mustard (ground)
*   30 ml vinegar (red wine)
*   30 ml Worcestershire sauce
*   5 g paprika
*   3 g crushed cinnamon
*   20 g celery salt
*   2 g black pepper

Directions:
*   On a 6 L electric pressure cooker, use the saute or browning mode.
*   Adjust the heat to medium and add the oil.
*   Brown the ribs in batches in heated oil; set aside.
*   Melt the butter in the pressure cooker.
*   When the butter has melted, add the leek.
*   Cook and stir leek for 2-3 minutes, or until soft.
*   Cook for 1 minute more after adding the garlic.
*   Fill the pressure cooker halfway with stock.
*   Cook for 1 minute, stirring constantly, to dislodge browned parts from the pan.
*   Click the Cancel button.
*   Combine remaining ingredients in a small dish; spread over ribs.
*   Return the ribs to the pressure cooker.
*   Close the pressure-release valve after locking the lid.
*   Set the pressure cooker on high for 40 minutes.
*   Allow the pressure to naturally release.

Nutrient value: Per serving
*   Calories: 232 kcal
*   Carbohydrates: 5 g
*   Protein: 20 g
*   Fat: 14 g

20. Slow-Cooker Chicken With Herbs

Prep Time: 5 minutes
Cook Time: 4 minutes
Servings: 4 people

Ingredients:
- 5 ml olive oil
- 10 g paprika
- 2 g garlic powder
- 2 g of seasoned salt
- 2 g dried thyme
- 2 g dried basil
- 2 g black pepper
- Optional: 3 ml browning sauce
- 4 chicken breast halves, bone-in (150 g each)
- 120 ml chicken broth

Directions:
- Combine the first 7 ingredients plus, if preferred, browning sauce in a small bowl; rub over chicken.
- Fill a 5-quart slow cooker halfway with stock.
- Cook on low for 4-5 hours, or until the chicken is tender.

Nutrient value: Per serving
- Calories: 211 kcal
- Carbohydrates: 1 g
- Protein: 33g
- Fat: 7 g

21. Meat Tacos

Prep Time: 10minutes
Cook Time: 35 minutes
Servings: 6 people

Ingredients:
- 1.5 kg ground beef
- 2 big sliced onions
- 450 ml water
- 20 g chilli powder
- 3 g cumin,
- 20 g salt

- 2 g garlic powder
- 2 g crushed red pepper flakes

Directions:
- Cook beef and onion in a large cast-iron pan or Dutch oven over medium heat until meat is no longer pink; drain.
- Pour in the water and seasonings.
- Bring the water to a boil.
- Reduce the heat to low and cook, uncovered, for 15 minutes, or until the water has evaporated.

Nutrient value: Per serving
- Calories: 113 kcal
- Carbohydrates: 2 g
- Protein: 10 g
- Fat: 7 g

22. Roast Chicken By Mom

Prep Time: 15 minutes
Cook Time: 35 minutes
Servings: 6 people

Ingredients:
- 1 chicken broiler/fryer (2 kg)
- 8 g kosher salt
- 3 g coarsely crushed pepper
- 10 ml olive oil
- Optional: fresh thyme or rosemary, minced

Directions:
- Season the outside of the chicken with salt and pepper.
- Place the chicken on a rimmed baking sheet with a rack. Refrigerate overnight, uncovered.
- Preheat the oven to 220□ C.
- Remove the chicken from the refrigerator while the oven warms up.
- For 15 minutes, preheat a 12-inch cast-iron or ovenproof pan in the oven.
- Place the bird, neck side down, on a work surface.
- Cut through the skin where the legs meet the body.

- Thighs should be pressed down so that the joints snap and the legs lie flat.
- Place the chicken, breast side up, in a heated skillet; press the legs down so they lie flat on the bottom of the pan.
- Apply oil to the brush.
- 35-40 minutes, or until a thermometer placed into the thickest portion of the thigh reads 70°C-75°C.
- Remove the chicken from the oven and set aside for 10 minutes before carving.
- Before serving, sprinkle with herbs if desired.

Nutrient value: Per serving
- Calories: 405 kcal
- Carbohydrates: 0g
- Protein: 44 g
- Fat: 24 g

23. Tenderloin Of Pepper-Crusted Pork

Prep Time: 25 minutes
Cook Time: 30 minutes
Servings: 6 people

Ingredients:
- Dijon mustard, 45 g.
- 5 ml buttermilk
- 8 g fresh thyme, minced
- 5 g coarsely ground pepper
- 1 g salt
- 2 pork tenderloins (3 kg)
- 100 g soft bread crumbs

Directions:
- Preheat the oven to 215°C.
- Combine the first five ingredients.
- To construct a double roast, arrange tenderloins thick end to thin end, thick end to thin end, and tie together with kitchen string at 1-1/2-in. intervals.
- In a 15x10x1-inch pan, place on a rack.
- Cover with bread crumbs, pressing to adhere, then spread with mustard mixture.

- 30-40 minutes, or until a thermometer placed into the pork reads 65°C. (If necessary, tent loosely with foil to prevent overbrowning.) Allow to stand for 5 minutes.
- Remove the string before cutting into slices.

Nutrient value:
- Calories: 155 kcal
- Carbohydrates: 3 g
- Protein: 23 g
- Fat: 4 g

24. Rolls Of Club Turkey

Prep Time: 20minutes
Cook Time: 40 minutes
Servings: 4people

Ingredients:
- Trimmed 3/4 pound fresh asparagus
- 8 cutlets of turkey breast (450 g)
- 15 g Dijon-mayonnaise mixture
- 8 deli ham slices
- 8 provolone cheese slices
- 2 g chicken seasoning
- 2 g black pepper
- 8 strips bacon
- 100 g Dijon-mayonnaise mixture
- 20 ml of 2% milk
- 1 g chicken seasoning

Directions:
- Bring 1 L water to a boil in a big saucepan.
- Cook, uncovered, for 3 minutes, or until asparagus is crisp-tender.
- Drain the asparagus and immediately immerse it in freezing water.
- Pat dry after draining. Place aside.
- Spread Dijon-mayonnaise on the turkey cutlets.
- Layer ham, cheese, and asparagus on top.
- Season with chicken seasoning and pepper to taste.
- Wrap with bacon and roll up tightly.
- Cook the roulades in a large skillet over medium-

high heat until the bacon is crisp and the turkey is no longer pink, 12-15 minutes.

• Combine the sauce ingredients and serve with the roulades.

Nutrient value: Per roll

• Calories: 224 kcal
• Carbohydrates: 2 g
• Protein: 25 g
• Fat: 11 g

CHAPTER 18

RECIPES FISH

1. Halibut Blackened

Prep Time: 5 minutes
Cook Time: 20 minutes
Servings: 4 people

Ingredients:
- 20 g garlic powder
- 3 g salt
- 3 g onion powder
- 10 g dried oregano
- 3 g dried thyme
- 10 g cayenne pepper
- 3 g pepper
- paprika, 25 g
- 4 fillets of halibut (110 g each)
- 30 g melted butter

Directions:
- Combine the first 8 ingredients in a large shallow bowl.
- Add 2 fillets at a time, turning to coat.
- Cook fillets in butter in a large cast-iron skillet over medium heat until fish flakes easily with a fork, 3-4 minutes per side.

Nutrient value: Per serving
- Calories: 189 kcal
- Carbohydrates: 3 g
- Protein: 24 g
- Fat: 8 g

2. Mahi Mahi Grilled

Prep Time: 20 minutes
Cook Time: 10 minutes
Servings: 8 people

Ingredients:
- 100 ml teriyaki sauce (reduced sodium)
- 30 ml sherry (or pineapple juice)
- 2 cloves garlic
- 8 fillets of mahi mahi (130 g each)
- **Salsa of Fruit Tropical**
- 1 medium peeled and sliced mango
- 250 g chopped peeled and seeded papaya
- 75 g green pepper, chopped
- 120 g fresh pineapple, cubed
- 1/2 medium chopped red onion
- 60 g fresh cilantro, minced
- 60 g fresh mint, minced
- 10 g seeded jalapeño pepper, chopped
- 5 ml lime juice
- 2 g red pepper flakes, crushed

Directions:
- Combine the teriyaki sauce, sherry or pineapple juice, and garlic in a shallow dish; add the mahi mahi.
- Refrigerate for 30 minutes after turning to coat.
- Meanwhile, put the salsa ingredients in a large mixing basin.
- Refrigerate until ready to serve, covered.
- Marinade should be drained and discarded.
- Place the mahi mahi on a grill rack that has been

greased.
- Grill, covered, over medium heat for 4-5 minutes on each side, or until the fish flakes easily with a fork.
- With salsa on the side.

Nutrient value: Per serving
- Calories: 195 kcal
- Carbohydrates: 10g
- Protein: 32 g
- Fat: 2 g

---

3. Red Snapper With Crumb Coating

Prep Time: 10 minutes
Cook Time: 20 minutes
Servings: 4 people

Ingredients:
- 120 g toasted bread crumbs
- 30 g Parmesan cheese, grated
- 3 g seasoning (lemon pepper)
- 4 red snapper fillets
- 2 g salt
- 10 ml olive oil

Directions:
- Combine the bread crumbs, cheese, lemon pepper, and salt in a shallow basin; add the fillets, one at a time, and turn to coat.
- Cook fillets in batches in a heavy skillet over medium heat until fish just begins to flake easily with a fork, 4-5 minutes on each side.

Nutrient value: Per serving
- Calories: 288 kcal
- Carbohydrates: 9 g
- Protein: 36 g
- Fat: 10 g

---

4. Fillets Of Herb-Roasted Salmon

Prep Time: 5 minutes
Cook Time: 25 minutes
Servings: 4 people

Ingredients:
- 4 fillets of salmon (130 g each)
- 4 minced garlic cloves
- 15 g minced fresh rosemary or 15 g crushed dried rosemary
- 5 ml olive oil
- 10 g fresh minced thyme or 3 g dried thyme
- 1 g of salt
- 2 g black pepper

Directions:
- Preheat the oven to 220°C.
- Place the salmon, skin side down, in a greased 15x10x1-inch baking pan.
- Combine the remaining ingredients and sprinkle them over the fillets.
- 15-18 minutes, or until the salmon begins to flake easily with a fork.

Nutrient value: Per serving
- Calories: 301 kcal
- Carbohydrates: 1 g
- Protein: 29 g
- Fat: 19 g

---

5. Quick Salmon Patties

Prep Time: 10 minutes
Cook Time: 15 minutes
Servings: 3 people

Ingredients:
- 100 g finely chopped onion
- 1 big beaten egg
- 5 crushed saltines
- 2 ml Worcestershire sauce
- 1 g salt
- 1 g black pepper

- 1 can (400 g) drained salmon, bones and skin removed
- 30 g melted butter

Directions:
- Combine the first 6 ingredients in a large mixing bowl.
- Over the mixture, crumble the salmon and combine well.
- Form into 6 patties.
- Fry patties in butter in a large skillet over medium heat for 3-4 minutes on each side, or until firm and golden brown.

Nutrient value:
- Calories: 288 kcal
- Carbohydrates: 5 g
- Protein: 31 g
- Fat: 15 g

---

6. Fillets Of Seasoned Tilapia

Prep Time: 10 minutes
Cook Time: 15 minutes
Servings: 2 people

Ingredients:
- 2 fillets of tilapia (150 g each)
- 15 g melted butter
- 5 g Montreal steak seasoning
- 2 g flakes dried parsley
- 1 g paprika
- 1 g dried thyme
- 1 g onion powder
- 1 g pepper
- 1 g salt
- a pinch of garlic powder

Directions:
- Preheat the oven to 220°C.
- Drizzle butter over the tilapia in a greased 11x7-inch baking dish.

- Combine remaining ingredients in a small dish; sprinkle over fillets.
- Bake for 10 minutes, covered.
- Uncover and bake for 5-8 minutes, or until the fish begins to flake easily with a fork.

Nutrient value: Per serving
- Calories: 193 kcal
- Carbohydrates: 1 g
- Protein: 32 g
- Fat: 7 g

---

7. Kabobs Of Ginger-Tuna

Prep Time: 25 minutes
Cook Time: 5 minutes
Servings: 8 people

Ingredients:
- 16 cubes tuna steaks (450 g)
- 15 ml soy sauce
- 30 ml rice vinegar
- 15 g toasted sesame seeds
- 30 ml canola oil
- 3 g pepper
- 16 slices pickled ginger
- Optional: 1 bunch watercress
- 120 g mayonnaise with wasabi

Directions:
- Toss tuna with soy sauce and vinegar; chill for 30 minutes, covered.
- Drain the tuna and pat it dry, discarding the marinade.
- Sprinkle sesame seeds and pepper over tuna.
- Sear tuna in a big skillet until browned and the centre is medium rare or slightly pink; remove from skillet.
- Thread 1 ginger slice and 1 tuna cube onto each of 16 appetiser skewers.
- Place on a watercress-lined patter if preferred.
- With wasabi mayonnaise, serve.

Nutrient value: Per Piece
- Calories: 100 kcal
- Carbohydrates: 1 g
- Protein: 8 g
- Fat: 7 g

---

8. SALMON OVEN-ROASTED

Prep Time: 10 minutes
Cook Time: 10 minutes
Servings: 4 people

Ingredients:
- 1 (220 g) center-cut salmon fillet
- 5 ml olive oil
- 2 g of salt
- 2 g pepper

Directions:
- In a chilly oven, place a large cast-iron or other ovenproof skillet.
- Preheat the oven to 220ºC.
- Meanwhile, brush the salmon with olive oil and season with salt and pepper.
- Remove the skillet from the oven with care.
- Place the fish in the skillet, skin side down.
- Return to the oven and bake, uncovered, for 14-18 minutes, or until the salmon flakes easily and a thermometer reads 60°C.
- Cut the salmon into four equal pieces.

Nutrient value: Per serving
- Calories: 295 kcal
- Carbohydrates: 0g
- Protein: 29g
- Fat: 19 g

---

9. CITRUS SALMON EN PAPILLOTE

Prep Time: 20 minutes
Cook Time: 15 minuteS
Servings: 6 people
Ingredients:

- 6 orange wedges
- 6 lime wedges
- 6 fillets of salmon (110 g)
- 450 g fresh asparagus, trimmed and cut in half
- Cooking spray scented with olive oil
- 2 g of salt
- 1 g pepper
- 30 g fresh parsley, minced
- 45 ml lemon juice

Directions:
- Preheat the oven to 220°C.
- Fold six 15x10-inch pieces of parchment or heavy-duty foil in half. Place a citrus slice on one side of each piece.
- Serve with fish and asparagus on top.
- Spritz the pan with cooking spray.
- Season with salt, pepper, and parsley to taste.
- Drizzle with lemon juice if desired.
- Fold the paper over the fish and crimp the edges with your fingertips to produce firmly sealed packets.
- Place in baking dishes.
- 12-15 minutes, or until the salmon flakes readily with a fork.
- Carefully open the packs to enable steam to escape.

Nutrient value: Per serving
- Calories: 224 kcal
- Carbohydrates: 6 g
- Protein: 20 g
- Fat: 13 g

---

10. NUGGETS OF OVEN-FRIED FISH (COD FISH)

Prep Time: 10 minutes
Cook Time: 15 minutes
Servings: 4 people

Ingredients:
- 75 g of seasoned bread crumbs
- 75 g crumbled cornflakes

- 45 g Parmesan cheese, grated
- 2 g of salt
- 1 g pepper
- 600 g cod fillets, diced into 1-inch cubes
- Cooking spray scented with butter

Directions:

• Combine the bread crumbs, cornflakes, Parmesan cheese, salt, and pepper in a shallow basin.

• Coat the fish in butter-flavored spray before rolling it in the crumb mixture.

• Place on a baking sheet that has been sprayed with cooking spray.

• Bake for 15-20 minutes at 204°C, or until the fish flakes easily with a fork.

• Option 1: Cover and freeze unbaked fish nuggets on a baking sheet lined with waxed paper until hard.

• Return to the freezer in a sealed freezer container.

• Preheat the oven to 204°C before using.

• Bake the nuggets for 15-20 minutes on a rack on a prepared baking sheet, or until the fish flakes easily with a fork.

Nutrient value: Whole recipe
- Calories: 171 kcal
- Carbohydrates: 7 g
- Protein: 30 g
- Fat: 2 g

---

11. Cod Poached In Tomato Broth

Prep Time: 5 minutes
Cook Time: 15 minutes
Servings: 2 people

Ingredients:
• 450 g fillet of wild-caught fish, cut into 3-inch squares
• 250 g organic whole peeled tomatoes (BPA-free)
• 600 ml pastured chicken broth
• Saffron, just a pinch (about 15 threads)
• two bay leaves
• 45 ml avocado oil

to taste, sea salt

Directions:
• Heat the oil in a frying pan over medium heat.
• Crush the peeled tomatoes into the pan with your hands.
• To taste, add stock, saffron, bay leaves, and salt.
• Bring broth to a boil over medium heat, then reduce to a low heat.
• Cook for 5-7 minutes, or until the fish begins to flake, after adding the cod fillets.
• Serve the fish in a tomato broth.

Nutrient value: Per serving
- Calories: 167 kcal
- Carbohydrates: 1 g
- Protein: 18 g
- Fat: 10 g

---

12. Parchment Fish In An Air Fryer

Prep Time: 10 minutes
Cook Time: 15 minutes
Servings: 2 people

Ingredients:
- 140 g frozen cod fillets
- 60 g julienned carrots
- 45 g julienned fennel bulbs or 60 g julienned celery
- 75 g red peppers, thinly sliced
- 2 tarragon sprigs or 3 g dried tarragon
- 30 g melted butter
- 15 ml lemon juice
- 10 g kosher salt, divided
- 15 ml oil
- 2 g ground black pepper

Directions:
• Melted butter, tarragon, 2 g salt, and lemon juice in a medium mixing bowl
• Mix until you have a creamy sauce.
• Mix in the julienned vegetables thoroughly. Place aside.

- Cut two parchment squares large enough to hold the fish and vegetables.
- Spray the fish fillets with oil and season both sides with salt and pepper.
- Place one fillet on each square of parchment paper.
- Half of the vegetables should be placed on top of each fillet.
- Any residual sauce should be poured over the vegetables.
- Fold the parchment paper over and crimp the sides to keep the fish, vegetables, and sauce inside the packet.
- Insert the packs into the airfryer basket.
- Preheat your airfryer to 176°C for 15 minutes.
- Place each packet on a platter.

Nutrient value: Whole recipe
- Calories: 251 kcal
- Carbohydrates: 8 g
- Protein: 26 g
- Fat: 12 g

---

13. CAKES OF KETO FISH WITH DRIPPING SAUCE

Prep Time: 5 minutes
Cook Time: 10 minutes
Servings: 6 people

Ingredients:
- 450 g raw boneless white fish (preferably local and wild caught)
- 100 g cilantro (leaves and stems)
- a pinch of sea salt
- 3 g chilli flakes
- 1-2 cloves garlic (optional)
- For frying, use 10 ml coconut oil or grass-fed ghee.
- Avocado oil is a good neutral oil to use for hand lubrication.

INGREDIENTS FOR DIPPING SAUCE:

- 2 avocados, ripe
- 1 lemon, freshly squeezed
- a pinch of sea salt
- 10 ml water

Directions:
- Combine the fish, herbs, garlic (if using), salt, chile, and fish in a food processor. Blitz until everything is evenly blended.
- Add coconut oil or ghee to a large frying pan over medium-high heat and stir to coat.
- Roll the fish mixture into 6 patties with oiled hands.
- Place the cakes in the hot frying pan.
- Cook until golden brown and cooked thoroughly on both sides.
- While the fish cakes are frying, combine all of the dipping sauce ingredients (beginning with the lemon juice) in a small food processor or blender and puree until smooth and creamy.
- If desired, add more lemon juice or salt to the mixture.
- When the fish cakes are done, serve them warm with a dipping sauce.

Nutrient value: Per Serving
- Calories: 69 kcal
- Carbohydrates: 2 g
- Protein: 2 g
- Fat: 6 g

---

14. SKILLET BUTTERED COD FISH

Prep Time: 5 minutes
Cook Time: 5 minutes
Servings: 4 people

Ingredients:
- 350 g cod fillets
- 90 g sliced unsalted butter

Seasoning:
- 1 g garlic powder

- 2 g salt
- 1 g ground black pepper
- 1 g ground paprika
- 3 g fresh herbs (parsley or cilantro)

a few lemon slices, drizzled with olive oil for dishing

Directions:
- In a small bowl, combine the seasoning ingredients.
- If desired, cut the fish into smaller pieces.
- Season the cod on all sides with the seasoning.
- In a large skillet over medium-high heat, melt 30 g butter.
- When the butter has melted, add the cod to the skillet. Cook for 2 minutes.
- Reduce the heat to medium.
- Flip the cod gently.
- Cook for another 3-4 minutes after adding the remaining butter.
- The butter will totally melt and the fish will begin to cook.
- (If you overcook the cod, it will get mushy and break apart.)
- Drizzle fresh lemon juice and herbs over the cod.
- Serve right away.

Nutrient value: Per Serving
- Calories: 294 kcal
- Carbohydrates: 5 g
- Protein: 30 g
- Fat: 18 g

---

15. Tandoori Salmon

Prep Time: 20minutes
Cook Time: 40 minutes
Servings: 4people

Ingredients:
- 100 g wild-caught salmon fillets
- 240 g sugar-free plain coconut milk yoghurt
- 15 ml unpasteurized apple cider vinegar
- 5 ml avocado oil
- 3 g powdered ginger or 1 inch piece fresh ginger mixed
- 3 g turmeric powder
- 3 g cardamom seeds, green
- 3 g cinnamon (Ceylon)
- 3 g ground cloves
- 3 g cumin seeds

RICE WITH CAULIFLOWER INGREDIENTS:
- 1 medium head riced cauliflower
- 5 ml coconut oil
- 1 spring onion, thinly sliced
- 1 sliced or spiralized tiny carrot
- 1 lime, cut into wedges 1/4 cucumber, sliced

Directions:
- Cook the tandoori salmon.
- Combine coconut yoghurt and all spices in a mixing basin.
- Cover the bowl with the fish. 30 minutes marinade (either on the counter if you plan to cook immediately, or in the fridge if cooking later).
- Preheat the oven to 176°C.
- Line a baking pan with aluminium foil.
- Remove the salmon from the marinade and place it, skin side up, on a baking sheet.
- Bake for 5 minutes at 176°C.
- Raise the oven rack to the top position and broil the salmon for 2-3 minutes, or until a light golden crust forms.
- Prepare the cauliflower rice while the salmon bakes.
- Heat the coconut oil in a large saucepan over medium heat, stirring to coat the pan.
- Place the cauliflower in the pan.
- Remove from heat after 3 minutes, or until softened.
- Divide the cauliflower rice over two plates, then top with the salmon.
- Garnish with the remaining vegetables and a squeeze of lime juice, if desired.

Nutrient value: Per Serving

- Calories: 432 kcal
- Carbohydrates: 18 g
- Protein: 34 g
- Fat: 23 g

---

16. Keto Fish With Parmesan Crust And Zoodles

Prep Time: 5 minutes
Cook Time: 10 minutes
Servings: 6 people

Ingredients:
- 90 g (divided) shredded Parmesan cheese
- 20 g fresh parsley, freshly chopped
- 100 g spiralized zucchini
- 60 g melted butter
- 450 g macadamias
- 400 g fillets of white fish
- 15 ml olive oil
- Salt, and freshly ground black pepper to taste

Directions:
- Melt the butter in a saucepan over medium-high heat and brown it.
- Meanwhile, roast the macadamia nuts for 2-3 minutes in a dry frying pan until brown.
- Remove from the pan and either smash using a mortar and pestle or finely chop with a knife. Place aside.
- On a plate, combine the parsley and half of the Parmesan.
- This produces the 'crust' mixture.
- Season the fish well with salt and pepper.
- Then, press all of the sides of the fish into the crust mixture.
- Make sure the fish is completely coated.
- Fry the fish in the same pan that you fried the macadamia nuts in, once the oil is hot. Depending on the size and thickness of the fillet, cook for about 2 minutes on each side.
- After frying one side and flipping the fish, add about a third of the browned butter to the pan and baste it with it.
- Remove from the pan and set aside to keep heated.
- Add the zoodles to the same pan, season with salt and extra browned butter, and cook for 30-40 seconds before turning off the heat.
- Place the zoodles on plates and top with macadamia nuts.
- Place the fish on top and top with the leftover browned butter and parmesan cheese.

Nutrient value: Per serving
- Calories: 659 kcal
- Carbohydrates: 2 g
- Protein: 46 g
- Fat: 56 g

---

17. Keto Thai Fish Curry And Bok Choy

Prep Time: 10 minutes
Cook Time: 20 minutes
Servings: 4 people

Ingredients:
- 15 ml coconut or avocado oil
- 30 g red curry paste
- 350 g coconut cream
- 250 ml of water
- 15 ml fish sauce
- 900 g white fish fillets, diced
- 450 g bok cabbage, thinly sliced
- Salt to taste

Directions:
- In a big saucepan, heat the oil, then add the curry paste and cook for 2-3 minutes on medium heat to activate the spices.
- Bring the coconut cream, water, and fish sauce to a boil.
- Reduce the heat after carefully adding the fish pieces.
- Cook for 10 minutes.
- Cook for 3-4 minutes more after adding the bok choy.
- Serve in big serving dishes.

Nutrient value: Per Serving
- Calories: 658 kcal
- Carbohydrates: 7 g
- Protein: 48 g
- Fat: 49 g

---

18. Green Sauce With Hake Fish

Prep Time: 5 minutes
Cook Time: 20 minutes
Servings: 3 people

Ingredients:
The green sauce
- 75 ml olive oil
- 12 avocado (100 g)
- 30 ml lemon juice
- 150 g fresh parsley cilantro, fresh
- 3 g garlic powder
- season with salt and black pepper to taste

Asparagus and hake
- 30 ml olive oil
- Green asparagus, 250 g
- 300 g boneless hake or cod fillets

Directions:
The green sauce
- In a blender or food processor, combine all of the ingredients and blend until the desired texture is obtained.
- We prefer it to be smooth and creamy.

Hake and asparagus
- Remove the rough section of the asparagus stem and wash it.
- Heat a tablespoon of olive oil in a frying pan large enough to hold the fish and veggies.
- Fry the asparagus for 6-7 minutes over medium heat.
- Season with salt and pepper to taste.
- While the asparagus remains in the pan, add the fish and cook for 2-3 minutes on each side.

- If necessary, add another tablespoon of olive oil for frying.
- Season with salt and pepper to taste.
- Stir the asparagus occasionally.
- Place the hake and asparagus on top of the sauce and serve.

Nutrient value: Per serving
- Calories: 470 kcal
- Carbohydrates: 5 g
- Protein: 35 g
- Fat: 33 g

---

19. Sesame-Crusted Tuna Steaks

Prep Time: 5 minutes
Cook Time: 10 minutes
Servings: 2 people

Ingredients:
Fried bok choy with garlic
- 10 ml mild olive oil or coconut oil
- 450 g bok choy, halved or savoy cabbage, quartered
- 15 ml tamari soy sauce

Tuna steaks with sesame crust
- 15 f sesame seeds (preferably a mix of white and black)
- 15 g almond flour, seasoned with salt & pepper
- 450 g fresh tuna fillets and steaks (1 per serving)
- 8 ml mild olive oil or coconut oil

Wasabi mayonnaise
- 60 g mayonnaise
- 10 g wasabi paste
- 10 ml lime juice

Directions:
Wasabi mayonnaise
- In a mixing bowl, combine the mayonnaise, wasabi paste, and lime juice.
- Place aside.

Fried bok choy with garlic

- Melt coconut oil and garlic in a large frying pan over medium-high heat. Fry the bok choy in the pan until it begins to turn colour.
- Turn the leaves over and drizzle with soy sauce.
- Continue to cook for a few minutes, or until the bok choy has softened slightly.
- Remove from the pan and set aside to keep heated.

Tuna steaks with sesame crust

- In a mixing bowl, add the sesame seeds, almond flour, salt, and pepper.
- Press the tuna steaks into the mixture on both sides until completely covered.
- Fry in a heated pan with coconut oil.
- We recommend merely cooking it for a minute on each side to keep it juicy and rare on the inside.
- Serve the tuna steaks with the bok cabbage and wasabi mayo on the side.
- Garnish with scallions, chiles, and lime wedges for a colourful display and a taste boost.

Nutrient value: Per serving

- Calories: 679 kcal
- Carbohydrates: 7 g
- Protein: 59 g
- Fat: 44 g

---

20. KETO ORANGE-CURED SALMON

Prep Time: 10 minutes
Cook Time: 20 minutes
Servings: 4 people

Ingredients:
Salmon cured

- 450 g boneless salmon fillets
- 1 orange, juiced and zipped
- 25 g salt
- 15 g pink peppercorns
- 250 g chopped fresh dill

Mustard mayonnaise

- 100 g unsweetened whole-grain mustard
- 30 ml cider vinegar
- 300 g mayonnaise
- 100 g whipping cream
- 350 g fresh dill, finely chopped
- 3 g salt
- 1 pinch ground black pepper

Directions:

- Make sure the salmon fillet is free of any little pin bones.
- Remove any leftover bones that may be seen along the thick back portion of the salmon with pliers or tweezers.
- Combine the orange zest, salt, and pink pepper in a small bowl.
- Reserve the orange juice.
- In a baking dish, place half of the dill.
- Rub half of the orange juice and half of the salt mixture into the skin side of the salmon, then place it in the baking dish on top of the dill mixture.
- Rub the flesh with the remaining juice and salt mixture.
- Distribute the remaining dill equally over the salmon.
- Wrap the fish with plastic wrap.
- A small cutting board should be placed on top of the
- Place a weight on top of the salmon, such as a large mortar or a jar of pickles, and make sure the weight completely compresses the salmon.
- Allow the salmon to cure in the refrigerator for two days, rotating it a few times before returning the weights on the meat.
- Scrape off all of the dill and orange when the fish is done.
- Using a paper towel, pat dry.
- Using a sharp, thin knife, cut the salmon into 0.8" (2 cm) thin slices on the bias (at about a 45-degree angle vertically).
- With a dollop of mustard mayo, serve the cured salmon.

Mustard mayonnaise

- Combine all of the ingredients in a small mixing dish.
- Season with salt and pepper to taste.
- Refrigerate for a few hours before serving.

Nutrient value: Per serving
- Calories: 785 kcal
- Carbohydrates: 5 g
- Protein: 25 g
- Fat: 73 g

CHAPTER 19

RECIPES SALADS

1. SALAD WITH CRISPY SPINACH

Prep Time: 10 minutes
Cook Time: 0 minutes
Servings: 2 people

Ingredients:
- 450 g spinach
- 1 chopped plum tomato
- 1 tiny apple, peeled and diced
- 120 g sliced cucumber
- 120 g cup shredded carrot
- 10 g pumpkin seeds
- 10 ml olive oil
- 10 ml balsamic vinegar

Directions:
- In a mixing bowl, combine the first five ingredients, then top with pumpkin seeds and drizzle with oil/vinegar.

Nutrient value: Whole serving
- Calories: 185 kcal
- Carbohydrates: 1 g
- Protein: 2 g
- Fat: 5 g

2. SALAD WITH A MINTY DRESSING FROM GREECE

Prep Time: 20 minutes
Cook Time: 0 minutes
Servings: 4 people

Ingredients:
- 1 small cucumber, diced
- 1 chopped red pepper
- 1 chopped green pepper
- 3 sliced plum tomatoes
- 3 sliced green onions
- 100 g crumbled feta
- 2 garlic cloves
- 45 ml olive oil
- 1-2 lemon juice
- 45 g chopped mint
- Season with salt and pepper to taste.

Directions:
- To create the dressing, combine the olive oil, lemon juice, mint, salt, and pepper in a mixing bowl. Place aside.
- Toss the remaining items in a basin with the mint dressing and serve.

Nutrient value: Per serving
- Calories: 200 kcal
- Carbohydrates: 5 g
- Protein: 9g
- Fat: 2 g

3. SALAD WITH ARUGULA

Prep Time: 10 minutes
Cook Time: 0 minutes
Servings: 4people

Ingredients:
- 250 g fresh arugula
- 1-2 finely sliced red onion
- 250 g fresh strawberries
- 10 g chopped pecans
- 10 ml olive oil
- 10 ml balsamic vinegar
- Season with salt and pepper to taste.

Directions:
- In a mixing bowl, combine all of the ingredients and drizzle with the oil/vinegar.
- Season with salt and pepper to taste.

Nutrient value: Per serving
- Calories: 150 kcal
- Carbohydrates: 4 g
- Protein: 7 g
- Fat: 12 g

4. CHICKPEA BOOSTER BOWL

Prep Time: 10 minutes
Cook Time: 0 minutes
Servings: 2 people

Ingredients:
- 50 g washed chickpeas
- 50 g shredded carrot
- 15 g sliced plum tomato
- 50g cucumber, chopped
- 20 g of red onion
- 15 g parsley
- 15 ml lemon juice
- Season with salt and pepper to taste.

Directions:

- Toss the ingredients together in a large mixing basin and serve.

Nutrient value: Per serving
- Calories: 150 kcal
- Carbohydrates: 10 g
- Protein: 19 g
- Fat: 15 g

5. HEART OF ROMAINE GRILLED

Prep Time: 10 minutes
Cook Time: 10 minutes
Servings: 4 people

Ingredients:
- 1 romaine heart, cut lengthwise
- 30 ml lemon juice
- Cherry tomatoes, 50 g
- 15 g Parmesan cheese
- 15 ml balsamic vinegar
- Season with salt and pepper to taste.
- 5 ml olive oil

Directions:
- Preheat the grill while coating the romaine halves with olive oil.
- Grill for 1 minute on each side (cut side down) on the grill.
- Serve warm, topped with the remaining ingredients.

Nutrient value: Per serving
- Calories: 100 kcal
- Carbohydrates: 6 g
- Protein: 14 g
- Fat: 7 g

6. TUNA SALAD

Prep Time: 10 minutes
Cook Time: 0 minutes

Servings: 1 people

Ingredients:
- 80 g tuna
- 200 g greens, mixed
- Cherry tomatoes, 30 g
- 20 g thinly sliced radish
- 1 sliced green onion
- 15 ml lemon juice
- 30 ml olive oil
- Season with salt and pepper to taste.

Directions:
- In a mixing dish, combine all of the ingredients and serve immediately.

Nutrient value: Per serving
- Calories: 210 kcal
- Carbohydrates: 14 g
- Protein: 29 g
- Fat: 25 g

---

7. SALAD WITH CHICKEN AND ASPARAGUS

Prep Time: 3 minutes
Cook Time: 4 minutes
Servings: 2 people

Ingredients:
- 50 g diced cooked chicken
- 100 g asparagus spears
- 50 g halved cherry tomatoes
- 10 g feta cheese
- 15 ml lemon juice
- 10 ml olive oil
- Season with salt and pepper to taste.

Directions:
- Bring water to a boil and cook asparagus tips for 3-4 minutes.
- Place in a bowl of ice cold water and strain.

Nutrient value: Per serving
- Calories: 220 kcal
- Carbohydrates: 10 g
- Protein: 22 g
- Fat: 15 g

---

8. SALAD OF WATERMELON AND ARUGULA

Prep Time: 5 minutes
Cook Time: 0 minutes
Servings: 2 people

Ingredients:
- 100 g diced watermelon
- 50 g arugula
- 20 g chopped red onion
- 20 g crumbled feta
- 15 ml balsamic vinegar

Directions:
- Serve immediately after combining the ingredients
- listed above.

Nutrient value: Per serving
- Calories: 110 kcal
- Carbohydrates: 2 g
- Protein: 9 g
- Fat: 5 g

---

9. SALAD OF CUCUMBER AND DILL

Prep Time: 15 minutes
Cook Time: 0 minutes
Servings: 4people

Ingredients:
- 100 g finely sliced cucumber
- 20 g chopped red onion
- 15 g coarsely chopped dill
- 15 ml olive oil
- 5 ml white vinegar
- Season with salt and pepper to taste.

Directions:
• Combine all of the ingredients and place in the fridge for 10 minutes before serving.

Nutrient value: Per serving
•   Calories: 80 kcal
•   Carbohydrates: 4 g
•   Protein: 9 g
•   Fat: 5 g

---

10. Salad Of Tomatoes And Basil

Prep Time: 5 minutes
Cook Time: 0 minutes
Servings: 1 people

Ingredients:
•   250 g halved cherry tomatoes
•   1 5 g basil, chopped
•   30 g minced red onion
•   15 ml olive oil
•   a drizzle of balsamic vinegar
•   Season with salt and pepper to taste.

Directions:
• Serve immediately after combining the ingredients.

Nutrient value: Per serving
•   Calories: 90 kcal
•   Carbohydrates: 3 g
•   Protein: 9 g
•   Fat: 3 g

---

11. Blt Chicken Salad

Prep Time: 10 minutes
Cook Time: 10 minutes
Servings: 8 people

Ingredients:
•   120 g mayonnaise
•   60 g bbq sauce
•   30 g coarsely sliced onion
•   15 ml lemon juice
•   1 g pepper
•   1 kg shredded salad greens
•   2 large diced tomatoes
•   350 g boneless skinless chicken breasts cooked and cubed
•   10 bacon strips cooked and crumbled
•   2 big hard-boiled eggs, sliced

Directions:
• Combine the first 5 ingredients in a small mixing bowl; stir well.
• Refrigerate until ready to serve, covered.
• In a large mixing basin, combine salad greens.
• Garnish with tomatoes, chicken, and bacon, and eggs if desired.
• Dressing: Drizzle with dressing.

Nutrient value: Per serving
•   Calories: 289 kcal
•   Carbohydrates: 5 g
•   Protein: 23 g
•   Fat: 19 g

---

12. Salad Caesar

Prep Time: 20 minutes
Cook Time: 15 minutes
Servings: 8 people

Ingredients:
•   450 g Parmesan cheese, shredded
•   2 g black pepper, finely ground
•   2 romaine hearts, peeled and sliced into bite-size portions (1.5 kg)
•   250 g halved grape tomatoes
•   100 g slightly crushed Caesar salad croutons
•   75 g Caesar salad dressing, creamy

Directions:
• Toss the cheese with the pepper in a small basin.

- Melt butter in a small nonstick skillet over medium heat.
- Spread 75 g cheese mixture evenly in a 6-inch circle in pan; cook, uncovered, until bubbling and rims are golden brown, 1-2 minutes.
- Remove skillet from heat and set aside for 15 seconds.
- Remove the cheese with a spatula and quickly drape it over an inverted 120 g. ramekin; gently press the cheese to form a bowl.
- Allow to cool completely. Repeat with the remaining cheese to make a total of eight bowls.
- Combine the romaine, tomatoes, and croutons in a large mixing basin.
- Drizzle with dressing and toss to coat just before serving.
- Arrange in Parmesan dishes to serve.

Nutrient value: Per serving
- Calories: 138 kcal
- Carbohydrates: 5 g
- Protein: 9g
- Fat: 9 g

---

13. SALAD WITH CHICKEN TACOS

Prep Time: 10 minutes
Cook Time: 3 hours
Servings: 6 people

Ingredients:
- 30 g chilli powder
- 3 g cumin,
- 3 g seasoned salt, and
- 3 g pepper
- 2 g white pepper,
- 2 g ground chipotle pepper, and
- 2 g paprika
- 1 g dried oregano
- 1 g crushed red pepper flakes
- 450 g boneless, skinless chicken breasts
- 250 ml chicken broth

- 1.5 g romaine lettuce
- Optional garnishes: Salad dressing of choice, sliced avocado, grated cheddar cheese, diced tomato or half cherry tomatoes, sliced green onions

Directions:
- Combine ingredients and rub over chicken.
- Fill a 3-quart slow cooker halfway with water.
- Pour in the broth. Cook for 3-4 hours, covered, over low heat, or until chicken is cooked.
- Remove the chicken and allow it to cool somewhat. Using two forks, shred the chicken.
- Serve over romaine lettuce, with additional toppings as desired.

Nutrient value: Per serving
- Calories: 143 kcal
- Carbohydrates: 4 g
- Protein: 24 g
- Fat: 3 g

---

14. TARRAGON SALAD

Prep Time: 5 minutes
Cook Time: 5 minutes
Servings: 4 people

Ingredients:
- 175 g drained and shredded light water-packed tuna
- 250 g celery, chopped
- 75 g finely sliced sweet onion
- 100 g low-fat mayonnaise
- 30 g fresh parsley, minced
- 5 ml lemon juice
- 5 g fresh tarragon minced or 1 g dried tarragon
- 2 g Dijon mustard
- 1 g ground white pepper
- Optional lettuce leaves
- Purchase Ingredients

Directions:
- Combine the tuna, celery, and onion in a small

bowl.
- In a mixing bowl, combine the mayonnaise, parsley, lemon juice, tarragon, mustard, and pepper.
- Serve on lettuce leaves if desired.

Nutrient value: Per serving
- Calories: 151 kcal
- Carbohydrates: 4 g
- Protein: 17 g
- Fat: 7 g

---

15. SKILLET CABBAGE SALAD

Prep Time: 10 minutes
Cook Time: 15 minutes
Servings: 6 people

Ingredients:
- 10 g melted butter
- 1 Kg cabbage, shredded
- 1 green pepper, thinly sliced
- 30 ml water
- 2 g salt
- 1 g pepper
- 75 g softened and diced cream cheese

Directions:
- In a large cast-iron or other heavy skillet, melt the butter; add the cabbage and green pepper and toss to coat.
- Mix in the water, salt, and pepper.
- Cover and cook for 8-10 minutes, or until the cabbage is soft.
- Stir in the cream cheese until it is melted.

Nutrient value: Per serving
- Calories: 100 kcal
- Carbohydrates: 4 g
- Protein: 2 g
- Fat: 9 g

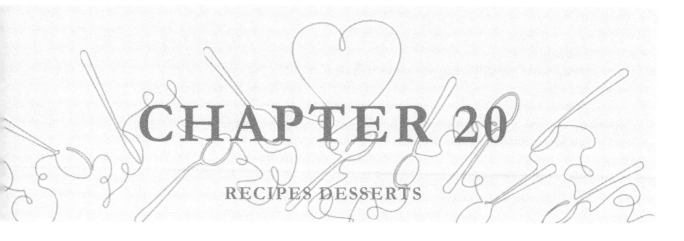

CHAPTER 20

RECIPES DESSERTS

1. COFFEE EGG FAST CUSTARD PUDDING

Prep Time: 5minutes
Cook Time: 15minutes
Servings: 4people

Ingredients:
- 120 g mascarpone cheese
- 60 g butter unsalted
- 5 g instant espresso powder
- 4 large eggs separated
- 3 g Sweet Leaf stevia drops
- 2 g monk fruit liquid extract
- 2 g cream of tartar
- Xanthan gum or galactomannan powder, optional

Directions:
- In medium saucepan, melt together mascarpone cheese and butter.
- Whisk in espresso powder and egg yolks.
- Continue to cook on low heat, stirring occasionally until custard thickens.
- Remove from heat and stir in liquid sweeteners.
- Beat egg whites with cream of tartar until stiff peaks form.
- Gently fold egg whites into custard mix.
- Chill. If desired and beat in xanthan gum or galactomannan powder with an electric mixer to give more of a pudding consistency.

Nutrition fact: Per serving
- Calories: 300 kcal
- Carbohydrates: 1 g
- Protein: 8 g
- Fats: 3 g

2. PEANUT BUTTER CUP CHEESE CAKE

Prep Time: 20minutes
Cook Time: 50minutes
Servings: 4 people

Ingredients:
- The crust:
- 15 g butter
- 1 large egg
- 100 g almond flour
- 15 ml erythritol or xylitol
- 7 g cocoa powder
- The filling:
- 100 g cream cheese
- 75 g sour cream
- 1 large egg
- 30 ml erythritol or xylitol
- 1 ml vanilla extract or vanilla beans
- 30 g peanut butter
- The topping
- 15 g sugar-free dark chocolate
- 10 ml coconut oil

Directions:

- Chocolate crust:
- Preheat oven to 150°C using the convection setting.
- Melt the butter and mix with all the other ingredients for the crust in a medium-sized bowl.
- Spread the mixture in the bottom of a 23 cm spring form pan.
- Bake for 10 minutes, remove and let cool at room temperature.
- Peanut butter filling
- Increase oven temperature to 200°C using the convection setting.
- Mix cream cheese softened at room temperature, sour cream and eggs until smooth.
- Add sweetener, vanilla extract, peanut butter and mix until incorporated.
- Pour the filling over the bottom and tap the form gently against the counter to get rid of any air bubbles.
- Bake the cheesecake for 10 minutes.
- Lower the temperature to 100°C and keep baking for 25 minutes more.
- The cake should be wobbly but not liquid when shaking it gently.
- Turn off the oven but leave the cake in there with the door open for 2 hours.
- The topping
- Melt the dark chocolate and coconut oil in the microwave in 20 second intervals.
- Stir to combine. You can also use a double-boiler for this step.
- Pour the mixture over the cheesecake and place in the fridge for at least two hours to allow the cheesecake and chocolate to set completely.
- If you feel like garnishing the cake like we did you can use fresh flowers and edible gold dust. Make sure to use flowers that are safe to use in contact with food.

Nutrition fact: Per serving
- Calories: 344 Kcal
- Carbohydrates: 6 g
- Protein: 9 g
- Fats: 2 g
-

3. LOW CARB BROWNIE

Prep Time: 20 minutes
Cook Time: 60 minutes
Servings: 24 people

Ingredients:
- 175 g butter, softened
- 100 g almond butter
- 3 large eggs
- 60 ml erythritol
- 100 g cocoa powder
- 250 g almond flour
- 2 g baking powder
- 1 g salt
- 30 ml water
- 15 ml vanilla extract
- 2 g instant coffee powder (optional)
- 30 g dark chocolate with a minimum of 80% cocoa solids, chopped

Directions:
- Preheat oven to 175°C degrees.
- Line a 9 by 13 baking dish with parchment paper.
- Use a hand mixer or stand mixer to combine the butter, almond butter, eggs, and sweetener. Mix well until the sweetener is thoroughly incorporated.
- Add the cocoa powder, almond flour, baking powder, salt, water, vanilla extract, and instant coffee powder and stir until smooth.
- Lightly mix in the chopped chocolate bar.
- Pour the mixture into the baking dish and smooth with a spatula.
- The batter will be thick.
- Bake for 25 to 28 minutes or until just set.
- Do not overbake or the bars will be dry.
- Let cool for 20 to 30 minutes before cutting.

Nutrition fact: Per serving
- Calories: 119 kcal
- Carbohydrates: 2 g
- Protein: 7 g
- Fats: 0 g

Prep Time: 5minutes
Cook Time: 13 minutes
Servings: 8people

Ingredients:
*   1 scoop protein powder of choice 32-34 g
*   250 g pumpkin puree can sub for banana
*   120 g smooth almond butter can sub for any smooth nut or seed butter
*   75 g cocoa powder
*   1 serving liquid stevia Optional
*   300 g chocolate chips of choice Optional

Directions:
*   Preheat the oven to 180ºC.
*   Line a small loaf pan with parchment paper and set aside.
*   In a mixing bowl, add all your ingredients and mix very well- The batter should be thick and smooth.
*   Pour the brownie batter in the lined pan and bake for 12-15 minutes, or until a skewer comes out just clean.
*   Allow brownies to cool in the pan completely.
*   For best results, refrigerate after for a further 2 hours.
*   Once cooled, cut into 8 pieces.
*   Either enjoy as is, or melt the chocolate chips of choice and dip each brownie in it until evenly coated.

Nutrition fact: Per serving
*   Calories: 126 kcal
*   Carbohydrates: 3 g
*   Protein: 8 g
*   Fats : 0 g

Prep Time: 1minutes
Cook Time: 1minutes
Servings: 1 people
Ingredients:

*   30 g butter, melted
*   1 egg, beaten
*   1 ml of vanilla extract
*   30 g almond flour
*   15 g coconut flour
*   30 g Swerve
*   10 g cocoa powder
*   2 g baking powder
*   pinch of salt
*   10 g sugar-free chocolate chips (optional)

Directions:
*   In a large coffee, add melted butter, egg, and vanilla and mix well.
*   Add the dry ingredients: almond flour, coconut flour, sweetener, cocoa powder, baking powder and salt.
*   Mix well.
*   Microwave on high for 55-60 seconds.
*   Be sure not to overcook, or the cake will be dry.
*   Optionally, top with sugar-free chocolate chips.

Nutrition fact: Per serving
*   Calories: 397 kcal
*   Carbohydrates: 5 g
*   Protein: 12 g
*   Fats: 1 g

Prep Time: 5minutes
Cook Time: 35minutes
Servings: 6 people

Ingredients:
*   2 Sugar free and fat free, instant pudding mix
*   4-5 Scoops whey protein powder
*   450 ml fat free milk
*   350 ml cold water

Directions:
*   Mix first 2 ingredients with spatula.

- Add milk and water slowly as you mix with an electric hand mixer on low setting for 2 minutes.
- Cover and put in refrigerator for at least 30 minutes before serving.

Nutrition fact: Per serving
- Calories: 110 kcal
- Carbohydrates: 9 g
- Protein: 15 g
- Fats : 0 g

---

7. PROTEIN WAFFELS

Prep Time: 5minutes
Cook Time: 10minutes
Servings: 5people

Ingredients:
- 3 eggs, medium-sized
- 30 grams almond paste , or other nut paste
- 25 ml coconut oil, liquid
- 45 g cottage cheese
- 60 grams protein powder
- 2 g cinnamon
- 1 g ground vanilla
- 2 g baking powder
- 50 ml erythritol

Directions:
- Mix all ingredients well in a blender or mixer to make homogeneous dough.
- Sweeten with erythritol to taste.
- Grease a waffle iron well and heat to medium heat.
- Pour 3-4 tablespoons of batter (depending on iron size) into the center and spread
- Close waffle iron and bake for 2-4 minutes.
- Do not open too early.

Nutrition fact: Per serving
- Calories: 167 kcal
- Carbohydrates: 5 g

- Protein: 15 g
- Fats: 3 g

---

8. CINNAMON SWIRL CAKE

Prep Time: 5minutes
Cook Time: 25minutes
Servings: 1 person

Ingredients:
- 75 g oats
- 1 egg white
- 1 scoop vanilla protein powder
- 10 g Stevia
- 7 g cinnamon
- 100 ml water

Directions:
- Preheat the oven to 165°C
- Blend the oats, egg white, and water until the consistency is smooth
- Pour the mixture into a bowl.
- Whisk it together with the protein powder and 5 g Stevia.
- The mixture should be like thick pancake batter.
- Pour half of the batter into a small nonstick pan and sprinkle with two-thirds of the cinnamon plus 5 g Stevia.
- Pour the remaining batter and sprinkle with the rest of the cinnamon.
- Pull a knife through the batter a few times to slightly mix in the cinnamon and Stevia.
- Bake for 25 minutes and let it rest for a few minutes before serving.

Nutrition fact: Per serving
Calories: 217 kcal
Carbohydrates: 13 g
Protein: 31 g
Fats: 2 g

Prep Time: 10 minutes
Cook Time: 34minutes
Servings: 4people

Ingredients:
- 4 large eggs, using only the yolks
- 300 g heavy whipping cream
- 10 g pumpkin pie spice
- 20 ml erythritol
- 2 ml vanilla extract
- Pumpkin pie spice, for serving

Directions:
- Preheat the oven to 180°C.
- Set aside one, 120 g oven-proof ramekin per serving, and a large baking dish with sides.
- Crack the eggs and separate yokes and the whites.
- Put the yolks in a medium-sized bowl for this recipe.
- You can store the egg whites in a small container in the refrigerator for another recipe if you wish.
- Add the heavy cream, pumpkin pie spice, sweetener, and vanilla extract to a small saucepan. Whisk together while bringing to a boil over high heat.
- Once boiling, remove it from the burner.
- Gradually add small amounts of the warm cream mixture into the egg yolks, whisking together until completely combined.
- Place the ramekins in the large baking dish and fill 3/4 of each ramekin with the cream mixture. Add water to the baking dish until it's about halfway up the sides of the ramekins.
- The water helps the cream mixture cook gently and evenly, for a creamy and smooth result.
- Bake on the middle rack for 25-30 minutes, or until the custard is set around the edges, and slightly jiggly in the center.
- Remove the ramekins from the baking dish and let cool.
- You can enjoy this dessert lukewarm or cold, preferably sprinkled with some pumpkin pie spice and a clementine segment on top.

Nutrition fact: Per serving
Calories: 286 kcal
Carbohydrates: 3 g
Protein: 9 g
Fats: 1 g

Prep Time: 5minutes
Cook Time: 10minutes
Servings: 4 people

Ingredients:
- 6 eggs
- 120 g cream cheese
- 90 g melted butter
- 100 g almond flour
- 100 g oat fiber
- 10 g baking powder
- 3 ml lemon zest
- 1 pinch salt (optional)
- 90 g fresh blueberries

Directions:
- In a bowl, whisk together eggs, cream cheese and melted butter.
- Mix the rest of the ingredients separately, except blueberries, and then pour into the egg mixture.
- Combine well until you get a smooth batter. Let rest for a few minutes.
- Fry the pancakes over medium heat in a small non-stick pan or cast-iron pan.
- Use around ⅓ cup batter per pancake.
- Fry for a few minutes and gently add some blueberries, without pressing them down too hard. Flip and fry for a few more minutes.
- Serve with whipped cream or browned butter.

Nutrition fact: Per serving
- Calories: 461 kcal
- Carbohydrates: 6 g
- Protein: 15 g
- Fats: 5 g

1. BERRY PROTEIN SMOOTHIE RECIPE

Prep Time: 5 minutes
Cook Time: 0 minutes
Servings: 6 people

Ingredients:
*   450 g Strawberries (hulled)
*   450 g Blueberries
*   450 g Raspberries
*   9 scoops ancient nutrition multi collagen protein powder
*   1 L can Coconut milk
*   100 ml Keto Simple Syrup (to taste)
*   15 ml Lemon juice

Directions:
*   Puree all ingredients in a blender, until smooth.
*   Adjust sweetener to taste as needed

Nutrition fact: Per serving
*   Calories: 230 kcal
*   Carbohydrates: 12 g
*   Protein: 15 g
*   Fats: 10 g

2. CINNAMON ROLL KETO SHAKE

Prep Time: 3 minutes
Cook Time: 2 minutes
Servings: 2 people

Ingredients:
*   220 ml milk or nut milk of choice
*   5 ml vanilla extract
*   15 g peanut butter powder
*   30 g cream cheese
*   20 ml granulated erythritol
*   15 ml sugar free maple syrup
*   10 g ground cinnamon
*   2 scoops bone broth protein powder
*   2 g kosher salt
*   250 g ice
*   whipped cream, ground cinnamon to garnish (optional)

Directions:
*   Add all ingredients to the blender, starting with just some of the milk if you like a thicker shake. Add ice and blend until smooth, adding more milk as you see fit.
*   Pour into a glass and top with whipped cream and a sprinkle of ground cinnamon.
*   Enjoy right away!

Nutrition fact: Per serving
*   Calories: 226 kcal
*   Carbohydrates: 10 g
*   Protein: 18 g
*   Fats: 5 g

3. Luscious Lime Smoothie

Prep Time: 5 minutes
Cook Time: 3 minutes
Servings: 2 people

Ingredients:
- 100 g cottage cheese
- 300 g Greek yogurt (4% fat)
- 75 g sour cream
- 75 g powdered erythritol or a few stevia drops (optional)
- 30 ml lime juice
- 30 ml lime zest

Directions:
- Place the cottage cheese in a blender or food processor and blend until smooth.
- Add the yogurt, sour cream, sweetener, lime juice, and lime zest.
- Blend until creamy.
- Pour the mixture into two serving glasses.
- Serve immediately.
- Garnish with additional lime zest, a lime wedge, or a dollop of freshly whipped cream.

Nutrition fact: Per serving
- Calories: 260 kcal
- Carbohydrates: 9 g
- Protein: 20 g
- Fats: 2 g

---

4. Shamrock Shake

Prep Time: 5minutes
Cook Time: 0 minutes
Servings: 1 person

Ingredients:
- 75 g vanilla protein powder of choice
- 450 g loosely packed spinach
- 75 g loosely packed fresh mint leaves
- 120 g mashed avocado or full-fat canned coconut milk
- 250 ml nondairy milk of choice

Directions:
- Add all ingredients to a high-powered blender and blend until smooth.

Nutrition fact: Per serving
- Calories: 362 kcal
- Carbohydrates: 5 g
- Protein: 24 g
- Fats: 0 g

---

5. Sugar Free Chocolate Smoothie

Prep Time: 5minutes
Cook Time: 0minutes
Servings: 1 person

Ingredients:
- 75 ml unsweetened almond milk
- 30 g Plain Greek yogurt
- 10 g no sugar added peanut butter
- 2 ml vanilla extract
- 10 g raw cacao powder or unsweetened cocoa powder
- 30 g collagen peptides
- 3 ice cubes
- 1 pinch sea salt
- optional: sugar-free sweetener to taste

Directions:
- Add all the ingredients to a blender and blitz for 1 minute until smooth.
- Taste and adjust sweetness to suit.
- Option to drizzle the glass with melted 90% dark chocolate for decoration.
- Storage: Best fresh.

Nutrition fact: Per serving
- Calories: 244 kcal
- Carbohydrates: 6 g
- Protein: 24 g
- Fats: 2 g

Prep Time: 5minutes
Cook Time: 0minutes
Servings: 1 person

Ingredients:

- 250 ml unsweetened almond milk
- 75 g heavy cream
- 1 scoop vanilla protein powder
- 100 g frozen strawberries
- Granulated or liquid stevia to taste (optional)

Directions:

- Place all the ingredients in a blender and blend until smooth.
- Serve immediately.

Nutrition fact: Per serving

- Calories: 358 kcal
- Carbohydrates: 14 g
- Protein: 20 g
- Fats: 8 g

Prep Time: 10 minutes
Cook Time: 0minutes
Servings: 1 person

Ingredients:

- 250 ml Unsweetened Vanilla Almond Milk
- 120 g Plain, Nonfat Greek Yogurt
- 100 g Roasted Beet Puree
- 30 g Chocolate Whey Protein Powder
- 10 g Unsweetened Dutch Processed Cocoa Powder
- 4 packets Natural Sweetener (stevia, Truvia, etc.)

Directions:

- Add the ingredients to a shaker bottle in the order the recipe is listed in (a blender works too!). Attach the lid, then SHAKE SHAKE SHAKE!

Enjoy!

Nutrition fact: Per serving

- Calories: 250 kcal
- Carbohydrates: 16 g
- Protein: 39 g
- Fats: 10 g

Prep Time: 5 minutes
Cook Time: 0minutes
Servings: 4people

Ingredients:

- 120 g heavy cream
- 250 g unsweetened almond milk, or coconut milk from the carton
- 1 medium avocado
- 30 g almond butter
- 30 g golden flaxseed meal
- 30 g cocoa powder
- 2 g cinnamon
- 2 ml liquid stevia, or to taste
- 1 g vanilla extract
- 1 g salt
- 8 whole ice cubes

Directions:

- Get your ingredients prepped pit and peel the avocado.
- Add all of your ingredients to a blender pulse together slowly until combined and then blend for 30-45 seconds until a smooth consistency appears.
- I recommend adding half the sweetener to the shake, tasting, and adjusting the sweetener to your taste.
- Once you have a smooth consistency, pour out into a glass and enjoy!

Nutrition fact: Per serving

- Calories: 453 kcal
- Carbohydrates: 6 g

- Protein: 8 g
- Fats: 2 g

Prep Time: 5 minutes
Cook Time: 0minutes
Servings: 1person

Ingredients:
- 1 ripe banana
- 1 scoop no sugar added vanilla protein powder
- 120 ml unsweetened vanilla almond milk
- 120 g cold or room temperature brewed coffee
- 300 g cubed ice
- Sprinkle of cacao nibs, for topping if desired
- 1 ml stevia extract, if desired

Directions:
- Add all ingredients except ice to a high powered blender and blend until mixed together.
- Slowly add ice to blender and process until creamy.
- Top with cacao nibs, if desired.
- Note: If you desire a bit of a sweeter shake, stir in 1 ml stevia extract.

Nutrition fact: Per serving
- Calories: 193 kcal
- Carbohydrates: 19 g
- Protein: 25 g
- Fats: 9 g

Prep Time: 5minutes
Cook Time: 0 minutes
Servings: 1person

Ingredients:
- 250 ml unsweetened almond milk
- 60 ml full-fat coconut milk or organic heavy cream
- 1 scoop Perfect Keto Chocolate Whey Protein powder
- 20 g cacao powder
- 2 ml liquid stevia to taste
- 5 g Perfect Keto Nut Butter or almond butter
- 3–4 ice cubes
- 10 g cacao nibs (optional)
- 30 g whipped cream (optional)

Directions:
- Add all ingredients to a high-speed blender, blending on high until smooth.
- Top with Perfect Keto Nut Butter or almond butter, cacao nibs, coconut flakes, or nuts if desired.

Nutrition fact: Per serving
- Calories: 273 kcal
- Carbohydrates: 4 g
- Protein: 17 g
- Fats: 0 g

CONCLUSION

Even a single human fasting cycle (e.g., overnight) will reduce the basal concentrations of many chronic disease-associated metabolic biomarkers, such as insulin and glucose. For example, many metabolic substrates and hormones patients need to fast for 8–12 hours before the blood draws to steady-state fasting levels. An important clinical and science issue is whether it is a viable and effective population-based approach to improve metabolic health to follow a normal, intermittent fasting regimen.

Also, intermittent fasting schemes aim to turn the positive effects of fasting schemes in rodents and other animals into realistic eating habits to reduce the risk of chronic disease in humans. Intermittent fasting schemes can be a positive solution to weight loss and metabolic health change for people who can comfortably manage periods of not eating or eating very little for several hours of the day, night, or weekdays. If proven to be effective, these eating regimes can deliver positive, non-pharmacological solutions to population-level health improvement with multiple benefits for public health.

How Intermittent Fasting Has Changed Me

My intermittent fasting experience is very good; otherwise, I would not have kept it (and still do) for so long. Personally, it has given me very good results both in body composition and improving my relationship with food. Of course, those results come over time, when it's part of your lifestyle-they aren't overnight changes.

If we talk about body composition, intermittent fasting added to training (especially strength training,) and a healthy diet, it has allowed me to maintain a good muscle mass level and reduce my percentage of body fat. In the times when I have strictly followed training and nutrition, I have managed to go down to approximately 16.5%; But, more importantly, in times when I have to reduce workouts for any issue, I have stayed without problems at around 20% without much effort and maintaining a good base of lean mass.

Regarding the relationship with food, intermittent fasting has helped me to notably reduce my anxiety when it comes to eating: knowing that I have established times to eat and that, within them, I eat when I'm hungry (without having to " wait for lunch or dinner ") has also made that anxiety to relax and learn to differentiate the" physical hunger "of the" emotional hunger ". I do not have the feeling at any time of "being on a diet", but of having some routines and sticking to them as part of my day today.

It is important to note two facts that have also been helpful to me whenever I have practiced intermittent fasting: on the one hand, the fact of being flexible, especially during weekends, when sometimes I do not comply with the same schedules as the days of diary. As I said above, it is important that the diet or, in this case, the nutritional strategy, adapts to us, and not us to it.

On the other hand, we have healthy diet most of the time with specific whims. Intermittent fasting is of little use, especially if we seek to improve our health through it if we base our diet on ultra-processed and other unhealthy products. Maintaining a healthy diet is essential if we want to achieve the benefits that this alternative promises us.

INDEX

Made in the USA
Monee, IL
07 August 2022